Complete Paleo Meals

A Paleo Cookbook Featuring Paleo Comfort Foods - Recipes for an Appetizer, Entree, Side Dishes and Dessert in Every Meal

Amelia Simons

ISBN-13: 978-1493773572

Table of Contents

Other Resources by Amelia Simons

Gluten-Free Slow Cooker: Easy Recipes for a Gluten Free Diet

Paleolithic Slow Cooker Soups and Stews: Healthy Family Gluten-Free Recipes

Paleolithic Slow Cooker: Simple and Healthy Gluten-Free Recipes

Going Paleolithic: A Quick Start Guide for a Gluten-Free Diet

4 Weeks of Fabulous Paleolithic Breakfasts

4 Weeks of Fabulous Paleolithic Lunches

The Ultimate Paleolithic Collection

4 MORE Weeks of Fabulous Paleolithic Breakfasts

Introduction

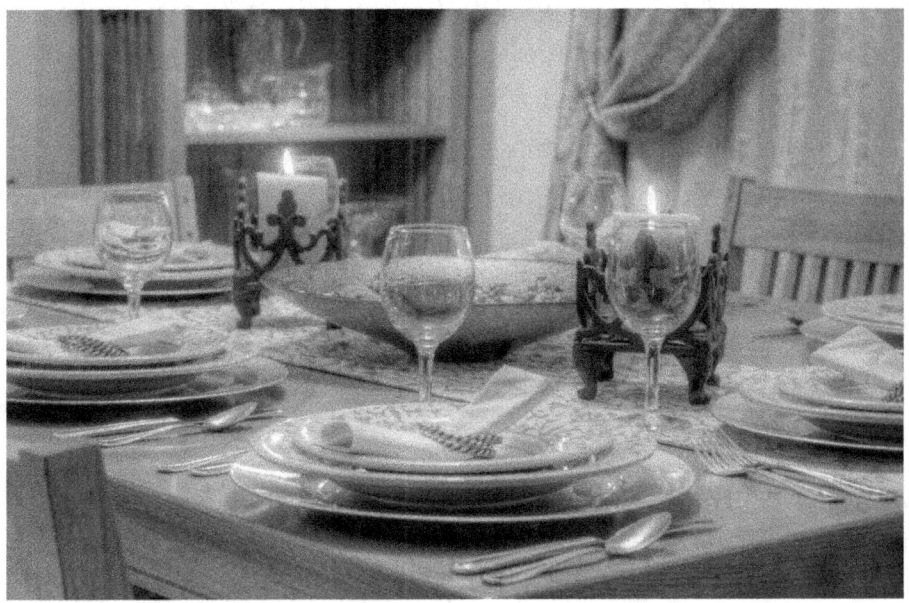

Having friends and family over to share a meal offers a chance to reconnect, plan, and make memories. We not only give a gift to others, but also to ourselves. Yet, with such busy lives as many of us lead, the thought of having people over can sometimes feel as though it is just "one more thing to do" and we miss out on the joy that comes with sharing a meal together.

Personally, I enjoy entertaining, yet for many, the planning and executing of a meal shared can be a challenge. Trying to figure out what to fix, organizing what to buy, and deciding in what order to prepare each dish so it all comes together are challenges many hosts and hostesses face. This is where ***Complete Paleo Meals*** comes to the rescue!

Complete Paleo Meals was written to offer you the help you need to enjoy having friends and family over. It has **12 totally complete meals**—one for every month of the year, for special occasions, or for times to make extras for leftovers. It is my way of giving you a guide that will make it easier for you to have friends over or to initiate a family gathering any day of the year. I have given you the tools to allow you to focus on other aspects of entertaining—like who to invite and how to decorate.

This is a unique cookbook for several different reasons:

1. Unlike most cookbooks, these meals are COMPLETE— from appetizers to desserts!

   - At the beginning of each meal, I list the names of all the recipe dishes

   - There is a GROCERY LIST of the main items you will need for each complete meal so you can copy it and take it to the store with you

   - Many offer a soup recipe you can serve as part of the meal or as an appetizer

   - You will find an entrée for each meal

   - All contain either a side dish and/or a salad, offering delicious ways to complement the entrée

   - Several offer delicious Paleo breads or muffins you can enjoy with your meal

- All offer scrumptious desserts to enjoy at the end of your meal—except for one, and that one has hot spiced cider instead. I do not know about you, but for me, that is just like dessert

2. As an added BONUS, I walk you through the PREPARATION PROCESS for every meal. For instance, I guide you through each meal's preparation by instructing you to do things like:

- Prepare some dishes the night before your gathering so they will have time to chill, etc.

- Alert you concerning certain dishes that need to be fixed first, progress to the next dish, then come back and finish up the first one so it can be finished when the rest of the meal is ready

- Put the menus in the ORDER you will be making them so you can see the FLOW of how the meal is prepared

- Offer helpful suggestions and give you "a heads up" when you need to know something specific about a recipe

Whenever you see this clock symbols, it concerns a time-sensitive issue or involves some special instruction.

- This cookbook contains recipes for meals that will serve 8 people. This means a family of four can easily invite another family of four over and you have just what you need. It also makes it easy to divide the ingredients by half if you only want to make a dinner for your family of four. Or, go ahead and make the whole meal for your small family and then you have leftovers for another dinner or lunch.

- What I have also tried to do is have several different dishes that allow you to serve your meal in courses—like they do in fine restaurants. Many have soups so you can serve this first and enjoy it. Then proceed to the main course and side dishes. And finally, top off your dining experience with a delicious dessert—right after or linger and visit for awhile and then serve it as a special treat.

- Just like my other cookbooks, I encourage you to buy the best ingredients you can afford when feeding your family and friends. While grass-fed beef and organic can be difficult, do what I encourage others to do—focus on *The Fabulous 14* and *The Terrible 20:*

The Fabulous Fourteen		The Terrible Twenty (Buy Organic)	
Asparagus	Mangoes	Apples	Lettuce
Avocado	Mushrooms	Blueberries	Nectarines
Cabbage	Onions	Celery	Peaches
Cantaloupe	Pineapple	Cherries	Potatoes
Eggplant	Sweet peas	Cucumbers	Spinach
Grapefruit	Sweet potatoes	Grapes	Strawberries
Kiwi	Watermelon	Green beans	Sweet bell peppers
**Genetically modified organisms (GMO) refer to foods that have been altered at the gene level. Because the health risks of consuming these foods have not been clearly identified at this writing, it is best to avoid eating them if possible.		Hawaiian papayas**	Sweet corn--white & yellow**
		Hot peppers	Yellow crookneck squash**
		Kale/Collard greens	Zucchini**

*This chart is based upon the information found in the book, *Rich Foods, Poor Foods* by Jayson and Mira Calton - ©2013

The Fabulous Fourteen are foods you can buy without having to worry very much about them being organic or any special labeling. However, with *The Terrible Twenty,* be sure to try to buy organic when you can find them, and afford them. Take special care to find out about the four products listed above concerning GMOs. Ask your local farmers and grocery workers to see if they were grown using genetically modified seed. Although many farmers that grow their crops organically, many do not realize they may be using GMO seeds.

Now it is time for you to make your way into this Paleo cookbook that I hope will help to build your confidence in your cooking skills and empower you to become a host or hostess extraordinaire!

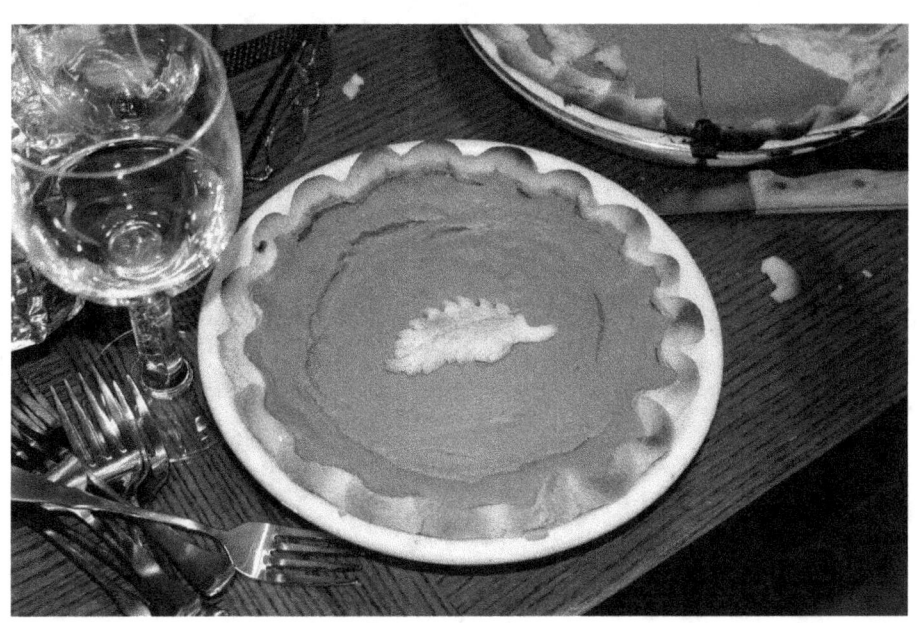

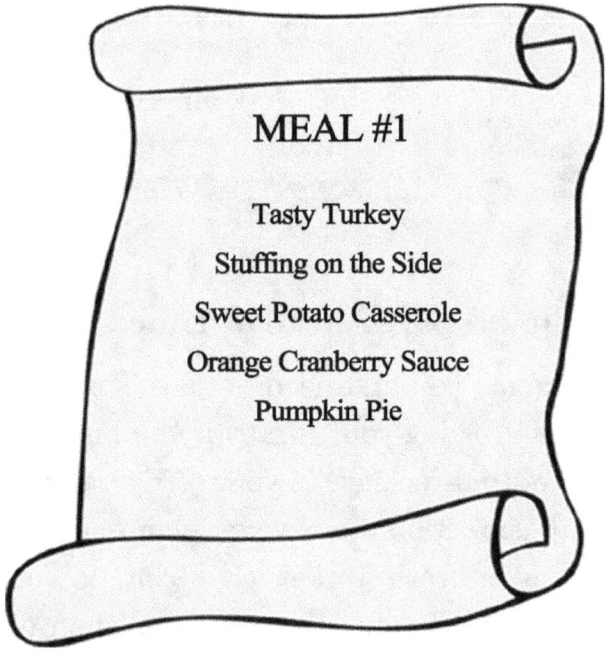

MEAL #1

Tasty Turkey

Stuffing on the Side

Sweet Potato Casserole

Orange Cranberry Sauce

Pumpkin Pie

Main Grocery Items (Foods like salt, pepper, staples and normal pantry items are not included)

Recipe ingredients have been **totaled** so you can see how much you will need for the entire meal (8 servings).

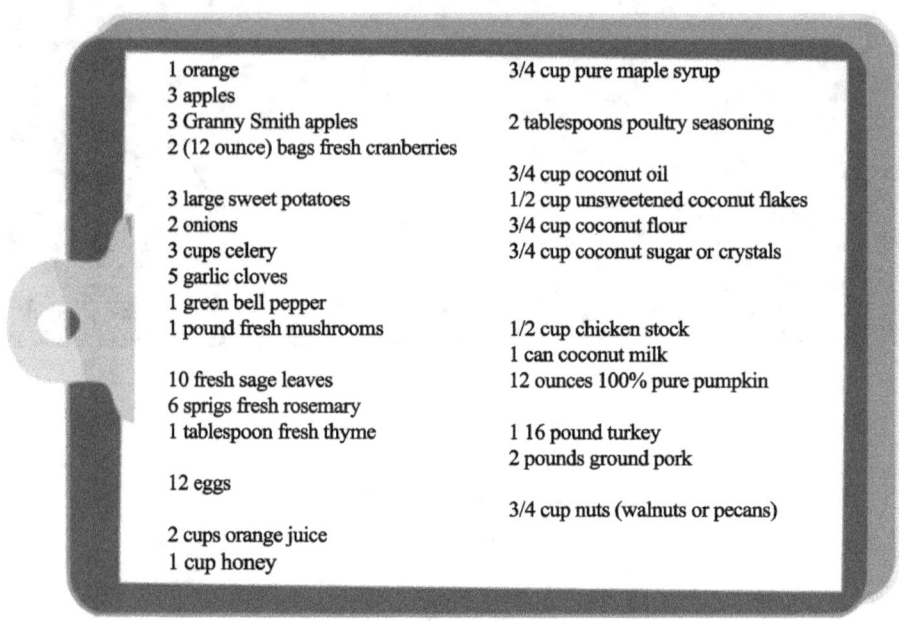

1 orange	3/4 cup pure maple syrup
3 apples	
3 Granny Smith apples	2 tablespoons poultry seasoning
2 (12 ounce) bags fresh cranberries	
	3/4 cup coconut oil
3 large sweet potatoes	1/2 cup unsweetened coconut flakes
2 onions	3/4 cup coconut flour
3 cups celery	3/4 cup coconut sugar or crystals
5 garlic cloves	
1 green bell pepper	
1 pound fresh mushrooms	1/2 cup chicken stock
	1 can coconut milk
10 fresh sage leaves	12 ounces 100% pure pumpkin
6 sprigs fresh rosemary	
1 tablespoon fresh thyme	1 16 pound turkey
	2 pounds ground pork
12 eggs	
	3/4 cup nuts (walnuts or pecans)
2 cups orange juice	
1 cup honey	

 Items to Prepare Ahead of Time

With this menu, you first need to make sure you follow the directions for defrosting your turkey if you buy it frozen. This may require two to three days in your refrigerator to defrost in time for you to cook it on the day you plan to eat it. You could consider buying a fresh turkey that can be found in the refrigerated section of your grocery store. Then defrosting is not an issue.

Additionally, you can make the cranberry sauce a day or two before, and prepare the pumpkin pie the morning of your party or the evening before as well. This will allow time for your cranberry sauce to chill thoroughly and for your pumpkin pie to set up and cool completely.

~~~~~~~~

Orange Cranberry Sauce

Ingredients:

- 1 teaspoon fresh orange zest (one orange should be plenty)

- 2 teaspoons freshly minced ginger

- 2 cups orange juice (fresh is great but from the carton will work, too)

- 2 (12 ounce) bags fresh cranberries

- 1 cup raw honey

Directions:

1. In a medium sized saucepan, place the orange zest and ginger

2. Add the orange juice and bring to a boil over medium-high heat

3. Once the mixture is boiling, carefully add the cranberries

4. Turn your flame down to medium and keep cooking the cranberries for approximately 10 minutes

5. Stir occasionally and continue to cook until the cranberries begin to pop open

6. When this occurs, remove your pan from the heat and add in the honey

7. Stir to help it melt and blend in

8. Allow the mixture to cool in the pan

9. Transfer the cranberry sauce into a serving dish, cover and refrigerate

10. Now it is ready for your party

~~~~~~~~~

Pumpkin Pie

Ingredients:

Crust:

- 2 teaspoons pure maple syrup

- 3 egg whites (room temperature)

- ¼ cup coconut oil, melted

- ¼ teaspoon sea salt

- ½ cup unsweetened coconut flakes

- ½ cup coconut flour

Filling:

- 3 whole eggs (room temperature)

- ¾ cup full fat coconut milk

- 1/8 cup pure maple syrup

- 1 teaspoon pure vanilla extract

- 1½ cups 100% pumpkin puree

- 1 tablespoon pumpkin pie spice

- ½ teaspoon sea salt

Directions:

1. Preheat your oven to 400 degrees F

2. Using a 9-inch spring-form pan (makes the pie easy to remove) or a regular pie pan, grease or spray the bottom and sides with coconut oil

3. In a medium mixing bowl, pour the maple syrup, egg whites, coconut oil, and salt and mix to blend

4. Now put the coconut flakes and flour into the bowl and mix completely so that no lumps are present

5. Pour the crust into your pan and press it out evenly across the bottom and pack firmly with the bottom of a flat measuring cup or glass

6. Place the pie pan into your preheated oven and cook for approximately 10 minutes or until it is slightly browned

7. Remove the crust from your oven and set aside to cool while you make the filling

8. Start this next step by LOWERING the temperature of your oven to 350 degrees F

9. Take a medium-sized mixing bowl and put in the eggs, coconut milk, maple syrup, and vanilla.

10. Using a hand mixer, beat for 1 to 2 minutes on HIGH to allow the eggs to be whipped

11. Add in the pumpkin, pumpkin pie spice, and salt

12. Once again, use your hand mixer to whip the filling on HIGH for 2 minutes

13. Gently pour the filling into your pre-baked crust

14. Place the pie into your preheated oven and cook for 30 to 35 minutes, making sure the middle does not giggle

15. Remove from the oven and allow to cool

One Other Thing to Do Before You Quit

Take a few minutes to peel, cut and boil the sweet potatoes for your Sweet Potato Casserole. Once you have finished boiling them for 20-25 minutes, just drain them, allow them to cool for 15-20 minutes, then put them in an airtight container and refrigerate them. This will save time when it comes to preparing them while the turkey is cooking.

 **On the Day of Your Meal**

Calculate how long you will have to cook your turkey using the formula consisting of the weight of your turkey times the number of minutes needed to cook each pound. Some directions give you guidelines like, "For 10-14 pound turkeys, cook _____ minutes/pound or _____hours." Once you know how long it needs to cook and the time you want to eat, you should have a good idea of when to start preparing it to go into the oven.

As a basic guide for deciding how big a turkey you might need, I usually calculate about 2 pounds of turkey for each person: 8 people x 2 pounds = 16 pound turkey.

~~~~~~~~

Tasty Turkey

Ingredients:

- 1 turkey (approximately 16 pounds)

- Coconut oil

- 1 apple, cored and quartered

- 1 small onion, peeled and cut in half

- 5-6 fresh sage leaves

- 5 sprigs fresh rosemary

Directions:

1. Preheat your oven to 500 degrees F (No, you read this correctly) and place the shelf your turkey will bake on at the bottom of your oven

2. Remove any innards packaged in the cavity of the turkey

3. Rinse it with cool water, then pat dry inside and out with paper towels

4. Place your turkey in a large baking dish that will accommodate your turkey, allowing for the accumulation of juices in the bottom. I like to line the bottom of my pan with foil

5. Taking your coconut oil, rub the outside of the turkey with the oil

6. At this point, you can sprinkle on some favorite seasoning or go on to the next step

7. Insert the apple, onion, sage and rosemary into the cavity of the turkey

8. Place the turkey into your hot preheated oven and allow it to bake at 500 degrees for approximately 30 minutes

9. At this point, LOWER the temperature of your oven down to 350 degrees F

10. If you have a meat thermometer or thermometer alarm, now would be the time to insert the probe into the breast where it is thickest. (If you have an alarm, you will want to know when it will reach an internal temperature of 160 degrees). Otherwise, cook your turkey for 2¼ hours to 2½ hours

11. Remove the turkey from the oven

12. Cover loosely with aluminum foil and allow it to rest for 15 to 20 minutes before you carve it

Gravy:

For a simple gravy, retrieve as best you can, the drippings from the bottom of the pan, pulse them in your blender or food processor and pour into a microwavable dish. You may need to heat up the gravy just before serving.

Next, Prepare Your Side Dishes

While your turkey is cooking, you will want to prepare your stuffing AND your casserole dish so that as soon as you take your turkey out of the oven to rest, you can immediately put these two dishes into your oven to cook while the turkey is cooling.

~~~~~~~~

Stuffing on the Side

Ingredients

- 2 pounds ground pork

- 1 tablespoon fresh thyme, chopped

- 1 tablespoon fresh rosemary, finely chopped

- 1 tablespoon fresh sage leaves, freshly chopped

- 1/2 teaspoon cayenne pepper

- 2 tablespoons coconut or olive oil

- 3 cups celery, chopped

- 5 garlic cloves, minced

- 1 green bell pepper, seeded and chopped

- 1 medium onion, chopped

- 3 Granny Smith apples, cored and chopped

- 1 pound mushrooms, chopped

- 3 eggs

- 1/2 cup chicken stock

- 2 tablespoons poultry seasoning

- Salt and pepper to taste

Directions:

1. In a large frying pan on your stovetop, add the pork, thyme, rosemary, and cayenne

2. Cook and brown completely

3. Set aside in a large mixing bowl

4. Now, in the same skillet, add your coconut oil and heat slightly

5. Add the celery, garlic, bell pepper, onion, apples, and mushrooms

6. Cook until the onions are translucent and the other vegetables and apple pieces are tender

7. Add these to the mixing bowl with the pork

8. In a small bowl, lightly whip your eggs, then add in the chicken stock and mix thoroughly

9. Pour the eggs over the pork and vegetables, add the poultry seasoning, salt, and pepper and stir completely

10. In a large baking dish that has been treated with coconut spray or oil, add the stuffing mix and distribute evenly

11. Cover with aluminum foil

12. Place the baking dish into your oven that should still be at 350 degrees F and bake for 25 minutes

13. Now uncover your baking dish and cook for 8 to 10 more minutes. This part is for helping to brown the stuffing

14. Remove when browned

Makes 8-10 cups

~~~~~~~~

Sweet Potato Casserole

Ingredients:

- 3 large sweet potatoes—peeled and diced

- 3 eggs

- 1/3 cup full fat coconut milk

- 1 tablespoon pure vanilla extract

- 3 tablespoons coconut oil, gently melted (warm, not hot)

- 2 apples--cored, peeled and quartered

- ¾ cup coconut sugar or crystals

- 1 teaspoon sea salt

Topping:

- 3 tablespoons coconut flour (break up lumps)

- ¾ cup walnuts or pecans, chopped

- ½ teaspoon ground cinnamon

- 3 tablespoons coconut oil, warmed to liquefy it

- 1/3 cup pure maple syrup OR coconut sugar (using coconut sugar will make mixture more crumbly)

Directions:

1. Preheat your oven to 350 degrees F

2. Place your sweet potato dices in a saucepan and cover with water

3. Bring water to a boil and boil the potatoes for 20-25 minutes or until the potatoes are fully cooked

4. Into a blender, add the eggs, coconut milk, vanilla, coconut oil, apples, coconut sugar, and salt and process until smooth

5. Once the potatoes are cooked, add them to a large mixing bowl and mash them

6. Now add the mixture from the blender to the mashed potatoes and mix completely

7. Using a greased baking dish (about 9-inch x 9-inch), pour the potato mixture into it

8. In a smaller bowl, make the topping by combining the coconut flour, nuts, cinnamon, and coconut oil and mix

9. Once these are combined, decide if you want to add a liquid sweetener (maple syrup) or a dry one (coconut sugar)

10. Place the topping over the potatoes

11. Baked in your preheated oven (uncovered) for 30 to 35 minutes or until your topping is nice and brown

You should now have enough food to feed 8 to 12 people, depending upon how many little ones you get to feed.

Note: The biggest challenge of this meal will be getting someone to slice the turkey while you finish up the side dishes. However, with at least 7 other people involved, surely there ought to be someone who can help you with this.

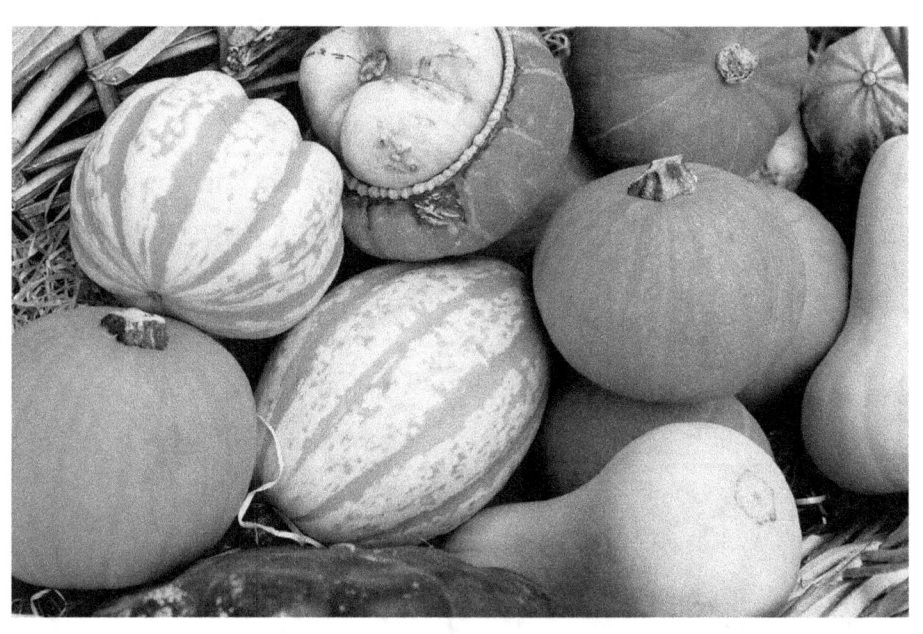

MEAL #2

Slow Cooker Aromatic Pork Loin

Apple Coleslaw

Bacon and Acorn Squash Patties

Cooked Apples

Pumpkin Gingerbread Muffins

Hot Spiced Cider

Main Grocery Items (Foods like salt, pepper, staples and normal pantry items are not included)

Recipe ingredients have been **totaled** so you can see how much you will need for the entire meal (8 servings).

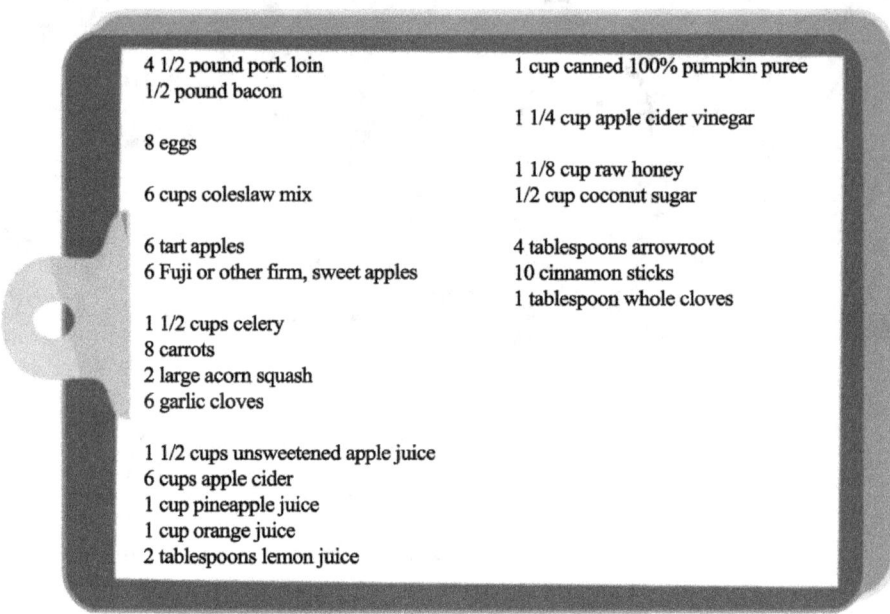

4 1/2 pound pork loin
1/2 pound bacon

8 eggs

6 cups coleslaw mix

6 tart apples
6 Fuji or other firm, sweet apples

1 1/2 cups celery
8 carrots
2 large acorn squash
6 garlic cloves

1 1/2 cups unsweetened apple juice
6 cups apple cider
1 cup pineapple juice
1 cup orange juice
2 tablespoons lemon juice

1 cup canned 100% pumpkin puree

1 1/4 cup apple cider vinegar

1 1/8 cup raw honey
1/2 cup coconut sugar

4 tablespoons arrowroot
10 cinnamon sticks
1 tablespoon whole cloves

Here is a meal that is tasty and not terribly difficult to prepare. With the main entrée cooked in the slow cooker, you will have time to fuss over other parts of your meal. Plus, you can even fix the Apple Coleslaw the day before and have it chilled completely before your meal, saving you time in the kitchen the day of your gathering.

## The Day Before Your Meal

Making the coleslaw ahead of time and allowing it to chill will meld the flavors for a great tasting dish.

Apple Coleslaw

Ingredients:

- 6 cups packaged coleslaw mix (bag of chopped cabbage found in the produce section) OR shred your own cabbage

- 6 unpeeled tart apples, chopped

- 1½ cups finely chopped celery

- 1¼ cup apple cider vinegar

- 3/8 cup raw honey (optional)

- 3 tablespoons olive oil

Directions:

1. In a bowl, combine the coleslaw mix, apples, and celery.

2. In a separate smaller bowl, whisk together the vinegar, honey, and olive oil.

3. Now pour the dressing over the coleslaw and toss together to coat the slaw.

If making this a day before, place it in an airtight container or a glass dish with plastic wrap over it and chill it overnight in the refrigerator.

 On the Day of Your Meal

Depending upon when your guests are going to show up, you will want to calculate when you want to start getting your pork ready for the crockpot. The pork loin takes about 6-7 hours to cook on LOW so if you put this in the crockpot early in the day, you might even be able to take a nap before guests show up!

Slow Cooker Aromatic Pork Loin

Ingredients:

- 6-8 carrots, cleaned and sliced (peeling is optional)

- 1½ teaspoons cinnamon

- ¾ teaspoon ground cloves

- ¾ teaspoon ground nutmeg

- ¾ teaspoon ground ginger

- ¾ teaspoon black pepper

- 6 garlic cloves, peeled and minced

- 1½ teaspoons sea salt

- ¼ cup coconut oil

- 4 - 4½ pound pork loin

- 2 cups water

Directions:

1. Turn your slow cooker on HIGH while you get your ingredients ready

2. Prepare a slow cooker by placing the sliced carrots in the bottom

3. Mix together cinnamon, cloves, nutmeg, ground ginger, black pepper, garlic and salt

4. Rub 1 tablespoon of the olive oil all over the pork loin

5. Now massage the spices over the pork loin

6. Place a frying pan on a high heat with the remaining olive oil in the bottom

7. Brown the pork loin on all side

8. Remove the pork and place it in the bottom of a slow cooker

9. Return to the frying pan on your stovetop and add the water to heat briefly

10. Now transfer the water from the frying pan to the slow cooker

11. Put the lid on the slow cooker and cook on HIGH for 3½ hours OR turn it down to LOW and cook for 6 hours

Makes 8-10 servings

About 2 Hours Before Your Meal

Now would be a good time to start cooking the acorn squash. Once it is fully cooked, remove it from the oven and allow it to cool so you can scoop out the cooked squash safely.

Prepare the ingredients for your cooked apple recipe and leave it in your saucepan. These will cook while you are frying your squash patties and while the muffins are baking.

About 1 Hour Before Your Meal

This is when you will want to prepare the patty mixture for frying. Once the mixture is combined, you will want to stop and fix the muffins and place them in muffin tins so they can cook while you are frying the squash patties

Bacon Acorn Squash Patties

Ingredients:

- 2 large acorn squash, cut in half with seeds removed

- 1/2 pound bacon, sliced into small pieces

- 1/4 cup coconut flour (break up any lumps)

- 2 teaspoons sea salt

- 1 teaspoon coarse black pepper

- 4 eggs

Directions:

1. Preheat your oven to 400 degrees F

2. Place your squash half face down on a cookie sheet that is lined with foil

3. Put the sheet into your preheated oven and cook until soft—approximately 30-35 minutes

4. As the squash is cooking, place your bacon slices into a large frying pan and cook

5. Once cooked, remove the bacon and set aside. Reserve the bacon drippings for later

6. When the squash is done and is cool enough for you to handle, scoop out the squash from its shell and place in a large mixing bowl

7. Add in your cooked bacon, coconut flour, salt, and pepper and mix thoroughly

8. In a small bowl, place the eggs and whip to combine thoroughly

9. Now add the eggs to the flour mixture and combine until thoroughly mixed

10. Heat up the bacon drippings in your pan

11. Once the drippings are hot, take a large spoon and scoop out enough mixture to make the size patty you want

12. Drop it gently into the frying pan and flatten with the back of a spatula

13. Continue placing patties into your frying pan until the mixture is used up. This may require a couple of batches

14. Cook each patty about 5 minutes on each side—until it forms a crunchy crust the way you like.

Makes 12-14 patties

~~~~~~~~~

Cooked Apples

These cooked apples are so delicious that we eat them for dessert at my house. We like them warm, right out of the pot. I have also mashed them up on numerous occasions so they are end up being like homemade applesauce. Either way, they are wonderful at the end of a meal.

Ingredients:

- 6 large Fuji or other firm, sweet apples—peeled and sliced

- 1½ cups unsweetened apple juice

- ½ cup coconut sugar

- 4 tablespoons arrowroot

- 2 teaspoons apple pie spice (optional)

Directions:

1. Place the apple slices in a medium to large saucepan

2. In a separate bowl, combine the apple juice, sugar, and arrowroot powder and mix thoroughly

3. Gently pour over the apple

4. Cover your saucepan with a lid

5. Over a low to medium flame, heat up the mixture

6. Cook the apples until desired tenderness— approximately 20 to 30 minutes, stirring occasionally

~~~~~~~~

Pumpkin Gingerbread Muffins

These moist and delicious wheat-free muffins are reminiscent of warm gingerbread cookies.

Ingredients:

- ½ cup coconut flour

- 2 teaspoons ground cinnamon

- ½ teaspoon ground nutmeg

- ½ teaspoon ground ginger

- ¼ teaspoon ground cloves

- ½ teaspoon baking soda

- ½ teaspoon baking powder

- ½ teaspoon salt

- 1 cup canned 100% pumpkin puree

- 4 eggs

- 2–3 tablespoons olive oil

- ¼ cup raw honey or pure maple syrup

- 1 teaspoon pure vanilla extract

- Pumpkin seeds or walnuts for topping (optional)

Directions:

1. Preheat your oven to 400 degrees F

2. Lightly oil your muffin pan with coconut oil or olive oil spray

3. In a medium-sized bowl, combine the flour, spices, soda, baking powder and salt

4. In another bowl, pour in the pureed pumpkin

5. Add the eggs one at a time, mixing well after each addition

6. Add the olive oil, honey, and vanilla and mix until blended

7. Combine the flour mixture into the pumpkin mixture and stir with a whisk until most lumps have disappeared

8. Take a large spoon and place equal amounts into your prepared muffin pan, filling each muffin about 2/3 full

9. Sprinkle the top of each muffin with a few seeds or walnuts if desired

10. Place muffin tins into your preheated oven and bake for 18-20 minutes or until a tester into the middle of a muffin comes out only with crumbs—not liquid batter

11. Allow the muffins to rest for a few minutes, then dump them out onto a wire rack to finish cooling.

~~~~~~~~

Now that your meal is cooked, you just have to slice your meat and enjoy.

When dinner is over, it is a great time to put together some hot spiced cider to enjoy while visiting with special family and friends. You can use a big coffee percolator or a big pot on your stovetop. While it is processing and heating up, it will fill your kitchen with deliciousness and invite your friends to stay awhile.

~~~~~~~~

Hot Spiced Cider

Spiced cider is something I thoroughly enjoy during the holidays but I have made it on several occasions when friends and family come over. I do not make it very often throughout the year because it is more of a cold-weather drink. It does include several fruit drinks so you do not want to drink too much of it, but it is a treat so give yourself permission to enjoy it occasionally. It is yummy!

Ingredients:

- 6 cups apple cider

- 1 cup pineapple juice

- 1 cup orange juice

- 2 tablespoons lemon juice

- 10 cinnamon sticks

- 1 tablespoon whole cloves

- ½ cup raw honey

- If you feel festive, thinly slice an orange and use it to decorate the side of your mugs

Directions:

Percolator method:

1. Pour in the apple cider, pineapple juice, orange juice, and lemon juice

2. Put the percolator stem and basket in place

3. Place the cinnamon sticks, cloves and honey into the basket of the percolator

4. Plug it in and wait for the little orange light to come on to tell you it is time to enjoy!

Stovetop method:

1. In a large pot, pour the apple cider, pineapple juice, orange juice, lemon juice and honey and stir to blend

2. Using a piece of clean cheesecloth, place the cinnamon sticks and cloves, tie closed and place it into the liquid

3. Over medium-low heat, cover the pot and allow the cider to heat up. You want to heat it slowly so the spice have time to work their way through the cider

4. Remove the cheesecloth and serve

Makes 8 (1 cup) servings

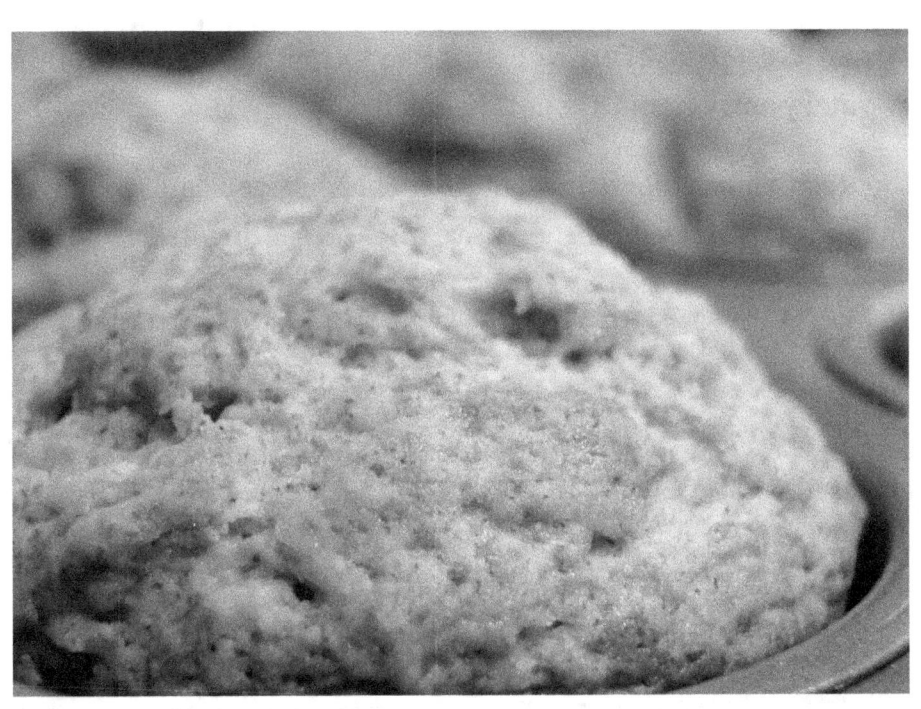

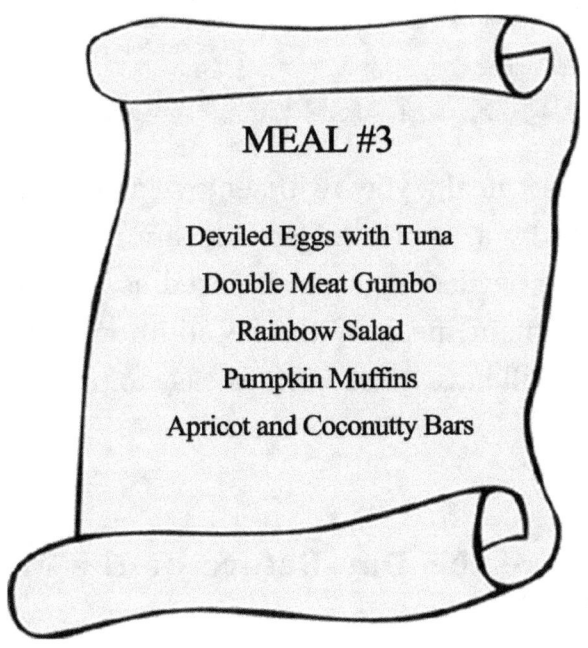

MEAL #3

Deviled Eggs with Tuna

Double Meat Gumbo

Rainbow Salad

Pumpkin Muffins

Apricot and Coconutty Bars

Main Grocery Items (Foods like salt, pepper, staples and normal pantry items are not included)

Recipe ingredients have been **totaled** so you can see how much you will need for the entire meal (8 servings).

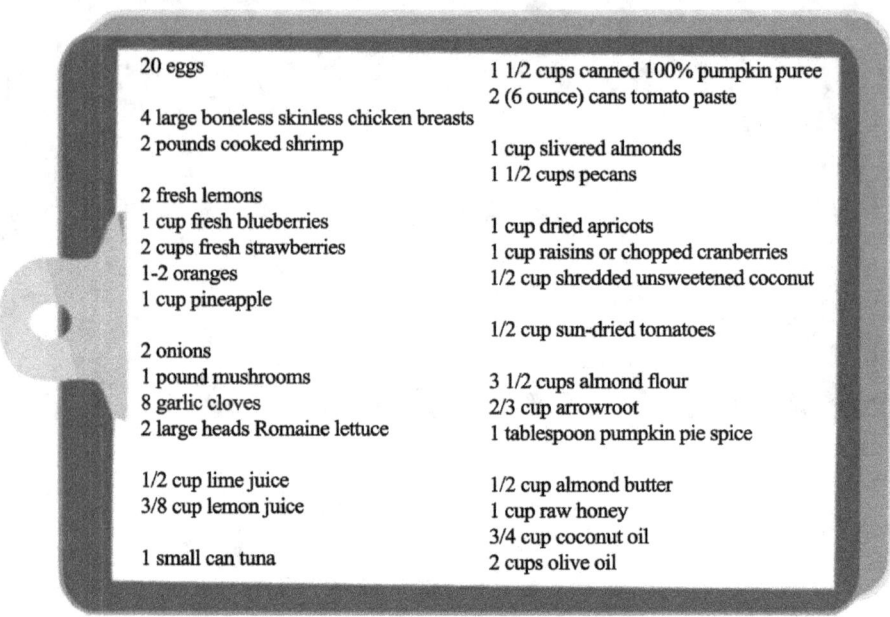

20 eggs

4 large boneless skinless chicken breasts
2 pounds cooked shrimp

2 fresh lemons
1 cup fresh blueberries
2 cups fresh strawberries
1-2 oranges
1 cup pineapple

2 onions
1 pound mushrooms
8 garlic cloves
2 large heads Romaine lettuce

1/2 cup lime juice
3/8 cup lemon juice

1 small can tuna

1 1/2 cups canned 100% pumpkin puree
2 (6 ounce) cans tomato paste

1 cup slivered almonds
1 1/2 cups pecans

1 cup dried apricots
1 cup raisins or chopped cranberries
1/2 cup shredded unsweetened coconut

1/2 cup sun-dried tomatoes

3 1/2 cups almond flour
2/3 cup arrowroot
1 tablespoon pumpkin pie spice

1/2 cup almond butter
1 cup raw honey
3/4 cup coconut oil
2 cups olive oil

With this meal, you will enjoy a delicious gumbo, accompanied by a colorful salad and muffins that round out the meal. The deviled eggs can be used as an appetizer or as part of your main meal. With the addition of the pumpkin muffins, you will have a meal that is easy to prepare and pretty to look at.

Prepare the Day Before or the Morning of Your Meal

Desserts often lend themselves to prior preparation so making the apricot coconut bars ahead of time will make for a calmer gathering. They will have plenty of time to chill, too.

Deviled eggs taste best (my opinion) when they have had time to chill in the refrigerator. In order for you not to have to rush making these, make them either the day before or early the morning of your gathering. I have also included a recipe for homemade mayonnaise for your eggs in case you do not have any one hand. Even if you do have some, you may want to make this first so you can include it in the deviled eggs. Believe me, it is worth the effort.

Deviled Eggs with Tuna

Ingredients:

- 1 dozen eggs, hard boiled, peeled and cut lengthwise

- 1 celery stick, finely diced

- ½ small onion, finely diced (about ¼ cup)

- 1 small dill pickle, finely chopped

- ¾ cup mayonnaise (homemade recipe below)

- 1 tablespoon spicy mustard

- ¼ teaspoon lemon juice

- 1 small can of tuna

- Salt and pepper to your liking

Directions:

1. In a medium mixing bowl, place the 12 yolks and mashed them up

2. Add the celery, onion, pickle, mayonnaise, mustard and lemon juice

3. Stir by hand to mix completely

4. Add in the tuna and season with salt and pepper to your liking

5. Carefully fill each egg white with the filling

6. Place in airtight containers and refrigerate until time to eat them

Makes 12 (2 eggs) servings

~~~~~~~~

How to Make Paleo Mayonnaise

Here is a recipe for Paleo mayo you can use over and over again!

Ingredients:

- 2 tablespoons fresh squeezed lemon juice

- 2 large eggs

- 1 teaspoon dry mustard

- Salt to taste. Start with 1 teaspoon

- ¼ teaspoon cayenne pepper (optional)

- 2 cups olive oil

Directions:

1. In a blender, add the lemon juice, eggs, dry mustard, salt, and cayenne (if using)

2. Pulse for a few seconds until the mixture becomes frothy

3. Turn your blender on a low setting and allow it to keep running

4. Slowly add the oil—almost a drop at a time—to the mixture until it begins to emulsify

5. Keep adding the oil slowly until it is all blended in

6. Add salt to taste

7. Store in a container in your refrigerator

Now with your deviled eggs tucked away in the refrigerator, it is time to make the dessert.

~~~~~~~~

Apricot and Coconutty Bars

Ingredients

- 1 cup slivered almonds

- 1 cup pecans

- ½ cup almond flour

- ½ cup coconut oil

- ½ cup almond butter

- ¼ cup raw honey

- 2 teaspoons pure vanilla extract

- ½ teaspoon sea salt

- 1 cup of dried apricots, chopped into small pieces

- ¼ to ½ cup of shredded unsweetened coconut

- Parchment paper

Directions

1. Preheat your oven to 350 degrees F

2. Place the slivered almonds and pecans on a cookie sheet and toast in your preheated oven for 8 to 10 minutes

3. Now place the toasted nuts into a food processor and pulse until they are coarse

4. Remove from the food processor and place in a medium bowl along with the almond flour and mix

5. In a microwaveable bowl, warm the coconut oil and the almond butter for about 20 seconds in the microwave until it has a fluid consistency when stirred

6. Stir in the honey, vanilla and salt into the almond butter mixture

7. Combine the flour mixture with the liquid almond butter mixture thoroughly

8. Add the apricot pieces and coconut and combine well OR you could use the coconut to coat the top of the bars

9. Lay parchment paper down in an 8 × 8 inch baking pan

10. Pat the mixture into the prepared pan with your fingers, making sure it is packed down well

11. Place in the refrigerator to harden or freezer for at least 1 hour

12. Cut into pieces and serve

On the Day of Your Meal

If you want to get your main dish ingredients ready ahead of time, I would suggest you cut up your chicken breasts into pieces and cook your shrimp. If you bought already cooked shrimp, you only have to rinse it under water in a colander for a few minutes before you add it to your gumbo.

Also, you could prepare your fruit by cleaning and cutting it up. You can combine the fruit together in a bowl but keep it separated from the lettuce and dressing until just before serving.

When you are getting closer to mealtime, prepare your muffin mix and then set them aside until about 45 minutes before you are going to eat. This will give them time to bake, cool in the tins, and still be served warm.

Pumpkin Muffins

Ingredients:

- 6 large – whole eggs

- 2/3 cup raw honey

- 1½ cups canned 100% pumpkin puree

- 3 cups almond flour

- 2/3 cup arrowroot

- 1 teaspoon baking soda

- 1 teaspoon baking powder

- ½ teaspoon sea salt

- 1 tablespoon pumpkin pie spice

- 1 cup raisins or chopped cranberries or a combination of both (optional, but oh so good)

Directions:

1. Preheat your oven to 350 degrees F

2. Lightly grease your muffin tins with coconut oil spray or rub with palm shortening or coconut oil

3. In a blender, place the eggs, honey, and pumpkin

4. Process and allow the blender to continue running while you mix your dry ingredients. This will add air to the eggs and help make them lighter and fluffier

5. In a medium to large mixing bowl, put the flour, arrowroot, baking soda, baking powder, salt, pumpkin spice, and raisins/cranberries and mix thoroughly

6. Pour the pumpkin mixture into the dry ingredients and mix until all ingredients are wet

7. Evenly divide the batter among the muffin tins

8. Place in your preheated oven and bake for 25 minutes. Muffins are done when they have started to pull away from the sides and the centers are no longer gooey

9. Allow the muffins to cool in the pan for about 15 minutes. Loosen and place on a cooling rack for them to finish cooling or serve warm

Makes 12-16 muffins

~~~~~~~~

Now that your muffins are ready for the oven, it is time to start cooking the gumbo. While it is cooking for those last 15 minutes, start to get your salad ready for the table.

Double Meat Gumbo

Feel free to add some extra spiciness to this dish if you like to enjoy gumbo dishes that kick!

Ingredients:

- ¼ cup coconut oil

- 2 onion, finely chopped

- 1 (16 ounce) package mushrooms, finely chopped

- 4 large boneless skinless chicken breasts, cut into bite-sized cubes

- ½ cup lime juice

- 3/8 cup lemon juice

- 1 teaspoon dried basil

- 1 teaspoon dried oregano

- 1 teaspoon dried thyme

- 1 teaspoon cayenne pepper

- 8 garlic cloves, peeled and minced

- 2 (6 ounce) cans of tomato paste

- ½ cup of sun-dried tomatoes

- 2 pounds cooked shrimp

Directions:

1. Place a deep frying pan over medium heat and add the olive oil to the pan

2. Place the chopped onion, mushrooms and the chicken cubes into the pan and stir

3. Add the lime and lemon juice, as well as the spices and garlic to the pan

4. Stir well and then cover with a lid and simmer for approximately 12 to 15 minutes, stirring occasionally

5. When the onions are soft and the chicken is cooked, stir in the tomato paste and dried tomatoes

6. Continue stirring until a sauce is created

7. Reduce the heat under the pan, and allow to cook for 10 to 15 minutes, stirring occasionally

8. Finally, stir in the shrimp and simmer

9. Once the shrimp is cooked, serve into bowls

~~~~~~~~~

Rainbow Salad

Ingredients:

- 2 large heads of Romaine lettuce, shredded or chopped

- 1 cup fresh blueberries

- 2 cups fresh strawberries, cleaned and sliced

- 1 cup fresh orange pieces, membrane removed if desired

- 1 cup fresh pineapple dices

- ½ cup chopped pecans

- Balsamic vinegar dressing or other favorite dressing

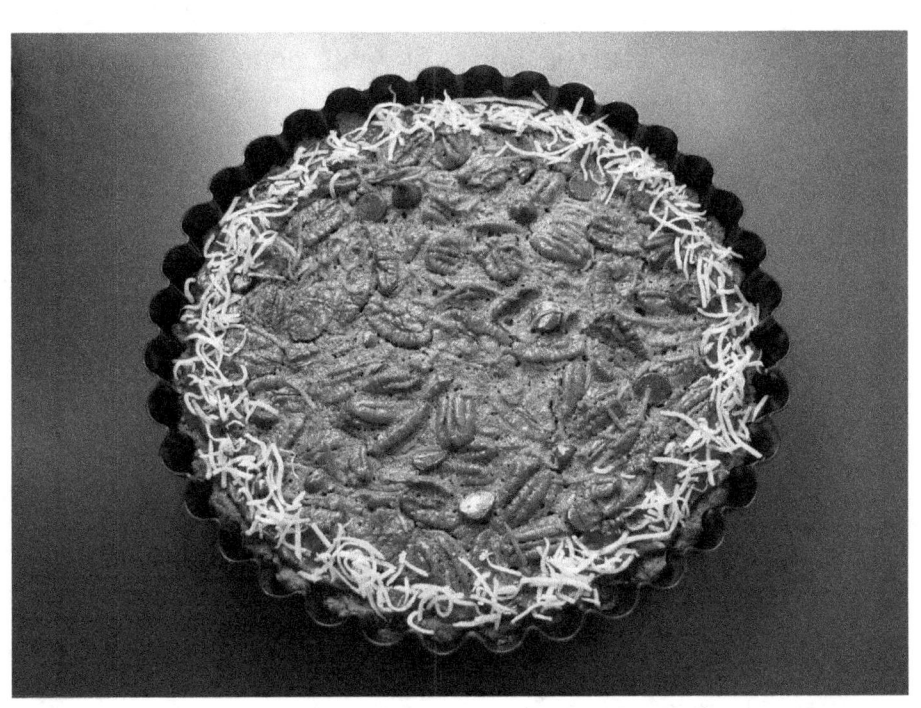

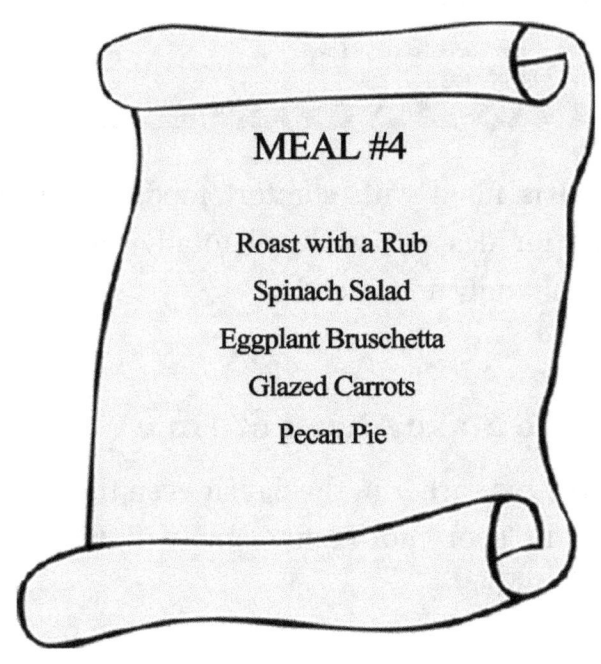

MEAL #4

Roast with a Rub

Spinach Salad

Eggplant Bruschetta

Glazed Carrots

Pecan Pie

Main Grocery Items (Foods like salt, pepper, staples and normal pantry items are not included)

Recipe ingredients have been **totaled** so you can see how much you will need for the entire meal (8 servings).

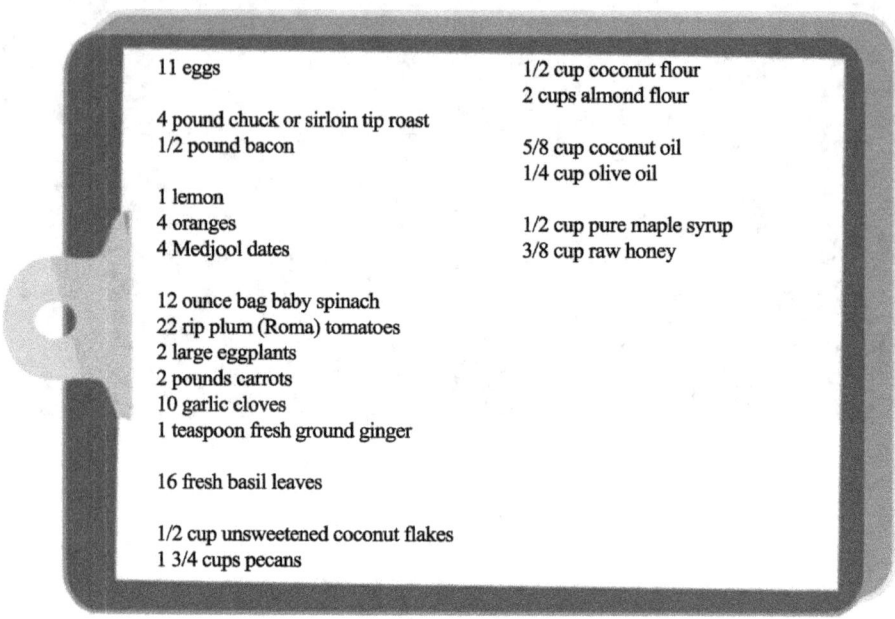

11 eggs	1/2 cup coconut flour
	2 cups almond flour
4 pound chuck or sirloin tip roast	
1/2 pound bacon	5/8 cup coconut oil
	1/4 cup olive oil
1 lemon	
4 oranges	1/2 cup pure maple syrup
4 Medjool dates	3/8 cup raw honey
12 ounce bag baby spinach	
22 rip plum (Roma) tomatoes	
2 large eggplants	
2 pounds carrots	
10 garlic cloves	
1 teaspoon fresh ground ginger	
16 fresh basil leaves	
1/2 cup unsweetened coconut flakes	
1 3/4 cups pecans	

This meal is filled with comfort foods. From a delicious roast, to pie for dessert, you will totally enjoy sharing this goodness with family and friends.

 **What to Make Ahead of Time**

Making the pie earlier in the day or even the day before will give it time to cool thoroughly and will make your meal preparations calmer.

Pecan Pie

Ingredients:

Crust:

- 2 teaspoons pure maple syrup

- 3 egg whites (room temperature)

- ¼ cup coconut oil, melted

- ¼ teaspoon sea salt

- ½ cup unsweetened coconut flakes

- ½ cup coconut flour

Filling:

- 1¼ cups pecans

- 1 tablespoon coconut flour

- 2 teaspoons of cinnamon

- Zest from ½ lemon or orange

- 4 Medjool dates—pitted, skin removed, and finely chopped

- ½ cup pure maple syrup

- 3 eggs (room temperature)

- 6 tablespoons coconut oil - melted

Directions:

1. Preheat your oven to 400 degrees F

2. Using a 9-inch spring-form pan (makes the pie easy to remove) or a regular pie pan, grease or spray the bottom and sides with coconut oil

3. In a medium mixing bowl, pour the maple syrup, egg whites, coconut oil, and salt and mix to blend

4. Now put the coconut flakes and flour into the bowl and mix completely so that no lumps are present

5. Pour the crust into your pan and press it out evenly across the bottom and pack firmly with the bottom of a flat measuring cup or glass

6. Place the pie pan into your preheated oven and cook for approximately 10 minutes or until it is slightly browned

7. Remove the crust from your oven and set aside to cool while you make the filling

8. In a food processor or coffee grinder, pulse 1 cup of the pecans (save the other ¼ cup of pecans to decorate the top later)

9. In a medium bowl, place the ground pecans, coconut flour, cinnamon, zest, and dates and stir to blend together

10. Now add the maple syrup, eggs, and coconut oil and blend until thoroughly combined

11. Pour this mixture into your precooked pie shell

12. Carefully place the remaining pecan halves on top

13. Place in the oven for approximately 30 to 35 minutes

14. Remove when fully cooked and allow to cool completely before slicing

On the Day of Your Meal

Prepare your roast by getting it rubbed down with the spices. You can safely allow it to come to room temperature before cooking (about 45 minutes) so it will remain be juicy.

Roast with a Rub

You just can't beat a great piece of meat with a delicious coating and this one gives you exactly that.

Ingredients:

- 1 teaspoon dried oregano

- 1 tablespoon sea salt

- 1 teaspoon garlic powder

- 1 teaspoon black pepper

- ½ teaspoon onion powder

- ½ teaspoon ground cayenne pepper

- 1 tablespoon paprika

- ½ teaspoon dried thyme

- 2 tablespoons olive oil

- 3 to 4 pound roast (chuck and sirloin tip work well)

Directions:

1. Preheat your oven to 350 degrees F.

2. Line a baking sheet with aluminum foil or use an oven safe Dutch oven

3. Begin by mixing the dry spices in a small bowl: oregano, salt, garlic powder, pepper, onion powder, cayenne, paprika, and thyme

4. Stir in the olive oil and make sure all the ingredients are blended thoroughly

5. Place the roast on the prepared baking sheet and then coat all the sides of the meat with the spice mixture

6. Roast 1½ - 2 hours in your preheated oven, or until the internal temperature of the roast reaches 145 degrees F

7. Allow the roast to rest for 15 to 20 minutes before slicing

Now that your roast is in the oven, it is time to prepare the eggplant. You will want to get it all ready and set it aside, then turn up the oven to 375 degrees F when you take your roast out and place it in the oven to cook.

Eggplant Bruschetta

Ingredients:

- 14 ripe plum (Roma) tomatoes

- 4 teaspoons apple cider vinegar

- 2 large eggplants

- 4-5 large eggs

- 4 cloves garlic, minced

- 16 fresh basil leaves, chopped

- 2 teaspoons paprika

- 2 teaspoons garlic powder

- 1 teaspoon sea salt

- 1 teaspoon black pepper

- 1 teaspoon dried thyme

- 2 teaspoons chipotle powder (optional)

- 2 cups almond flour

- 2-3 tablespoons coconut oil

Directions:

1. Preheat your oven to 375 degrees F

2. Once the tomatoes are peeled, cut them in halves or quarters and remove the seeds and juice from their centers

3. Also, cut out and discard the stem area

4. In a separate bowl, mix the tomatoes with the vinegar and set aside

5. Slice the eggplant into 8 round slices, each about ½ inch thick

6. Trim the skin, maintaining the round shape of the slices

7. In a small bowl, whisk the eggs

8. Mix dry ingredients and almond flour together and set aside in a separate small bowl

9. Grease a large baking sheet or pizza pan with olive oil

10. Dip the eggplant slices one at a time into the egg and then into the almond flour

11. One by one, place the coated slices in a single layer on the prepared baking sheet or pizza pan greased with the coconut oil

12. Top the slices with the tomato topping

13. Bake in the preheated oven approximately 15 minutes

14. Now change the oven setting to broil and continue cooking 3 to 5 minutes

15. Check the slices frequently during broiling to avoid burning

16. Remove from the oven when you are pleased with the brownness of your topping

~~~~~~~~

With the eggplant ready to go into the oven when the roast is done, now would be a good time to get your salad ready. Wait to add the dressing until just before serving.

Spinach Salad

Ingredients:

- ½ pound bacon, sliced in small pieces

- 12 ounce bag baby spinach (about 10-12 cups)

- 8 Roma tomatoes, diced

- ½ cup almond slices or pecans (optional)

- 1 orange—zested and juiced

- 2 teaspoons raw honey (warmed slightly so it flows easily)

- 2 tablespoons apple cider vinegar

- 2 tablespoons olive oil

- 1 tablespoon spicy brown mustard

- 3 garlic cloves, peeled and minced

Directions:

1. On your stovetop, cook the bacon slices until done

2. Drain on a paper towel and set aside

3. In a large bowl, place the spinach, tomatoes, and nuts and toss gently to combine

4. In a small container or bowl, mix the orange, honey, vinegar, oil, mustard, and garlic

5. Mix thoroughly

6. Pour on your spinach just before serving and mix to coat

Makes 8 servings

~~~~~~~~

With only one more dish to prepare, I have saved the easiest for last!

Glazed Carrots

Sometimes when I make this recipe, I like to use the shredded carrots that come in a bag in the produce section. Not only does this save some time in the preparation, but it makes for a beautiful presentation, too.

Ingredients:

- 1 teaspoon sea salt

- 2 cups water

- 2 pounds carrots, peeled and cut into 1/2" slices (or use shredded carrots)

- ¼ cup raw honey

- 2 oranges - zested and juiced

- 2 tablespoons coconut oil

- 1 teaspoon fresh ground ginger

- ½ - 1 teaspoon coarse black pepper

Directions:

1. In a medium to large saucepan on top of your stove, put the salt, water, and carrots and cook over a medium flame

2. Bring the water to a boil

3. Now cover, reduce the heat slightly and simmer for 10 minutes to allow the carrots to soften (If you are using the shredded carrots, they may be soft enough after 5 or 6 minutes)

4. Drain the water once the carrots are soft

5. Return the pan to your stovetop and add in the honey, orange juice and zest, coconut oil, ginger, and pepper

6. Stir together thoroughly as you cook your carrots over a medium flame for 4 to 5 more minutes. A glaze should start to form and thicken

7. Taste and season as desired with additional salt and pepper

8. Serve hot

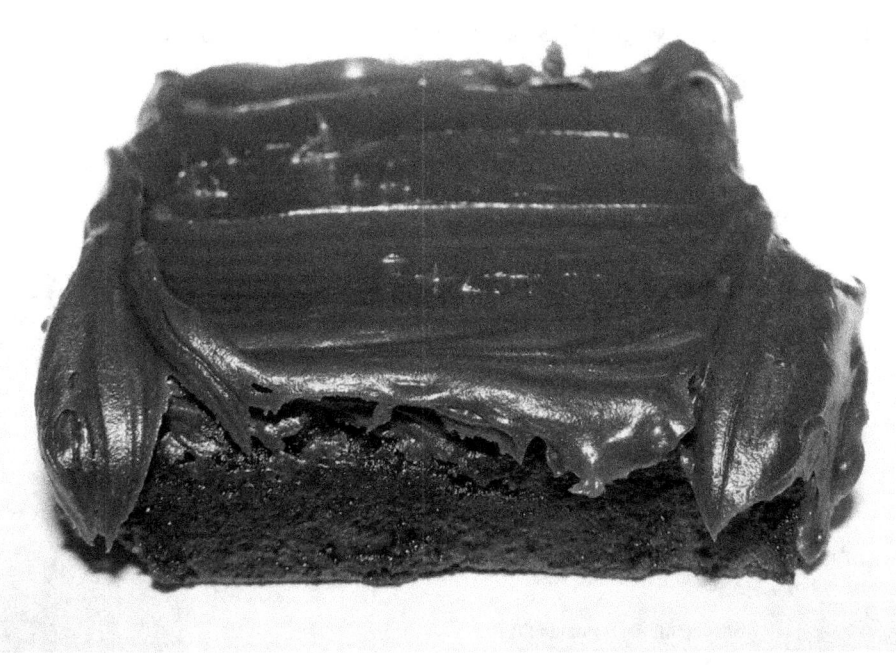

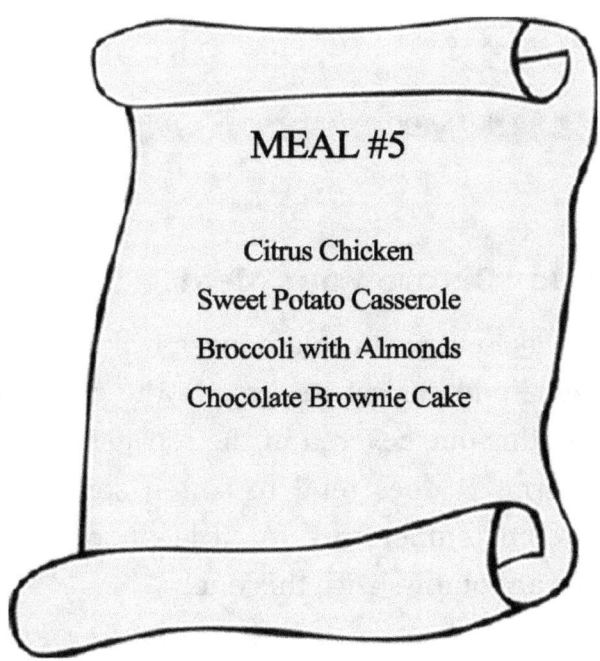

MEAL #5

Citrus Chicken

Sweet Potato Casserole

Broccoli with Almonds

Chocolate Brownie Cake

Main Grocery Items (Foods like salt, pepper, staples and normal pantry items are not included)

Recipe ingredients have been **totaled** so you can see how much you will need for the entire meal (8 servings).

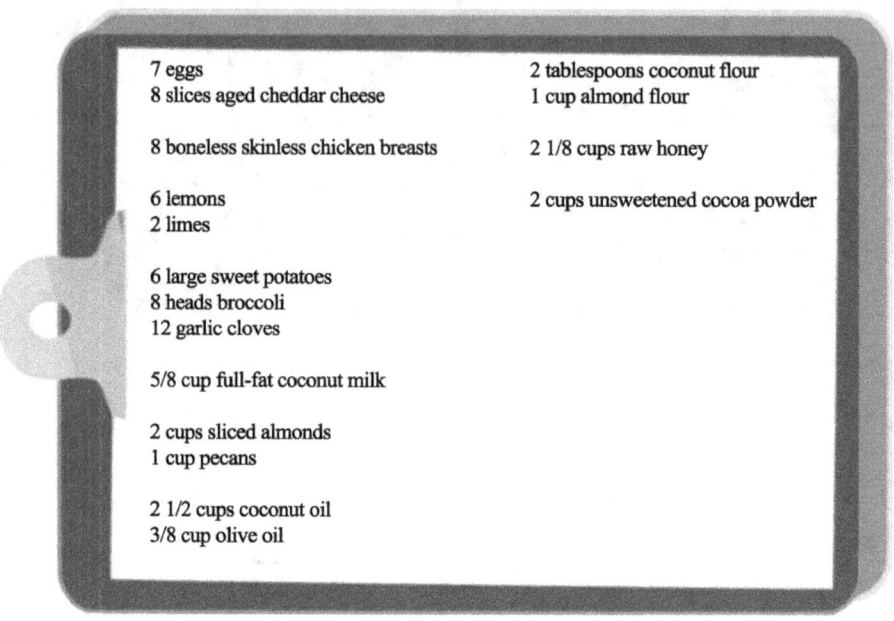

7 eggs	2 tablespoons coconut flour
8 slices aged cheddar cheese	1 cup almond flour
8 boneless skinless chicken breasts	2 1/8 cups raw honey
6 lemons	2 cups unsweetened cocoa powder
2 limes	
6 large sweet potatoes	
8 heads broccoli	
12 garlic cloves	
5/8 cup full-fat coconut milk	
2 cups sliced almonds	
1 cup pecans	
2 1/2 cups coconut oil	
3/8 cup olive oil	

 **The Day Before Your Meal**

Here is a cake every chocolate lover will adore. It is like a frosted brownie and easiest to prepare the day before. Make sure you keep this one covered in the refrigerator so the icing will remain firm. It does tend to soften somewhat when it remains at room temperature. A little bit of trouble, but I promise, you cannot miss with this one!

Chocolate Brownie Cake

Ingredients:

- 3 tablespoons coconut oil

- ¾ cup raw honey

- 2 teaspoons pure vanilla extract

- 1 cup unsweetened cocoa powder

- 1/8 teaspoon sea salt

- 4 eggs, beaten

Frosting:

- 1 cup raw honey

- 2 cups coconut oil

- 1 cup cocoa powder

- 1½ tablespoons full fat coconut milk

Directions:

1. Preheat your oven to 350 degrees F

2. In a medium-sized microwavable bowl, place the coconut oil and honey

3. Process in 20-second increments until the oil and honey are blended together. Do not make them hot!

4. To the bowl, now add the vanilla, cocoa powder, and salt

5. Stir to combine the ingredients

6. Now add in the beaten eggs and stir until a smooth consistency is achieved

7. Pour the batter into a square baking dish that has been lightly greased with coconut oil

8. Place the dish into your preheated oven and bake for 30 minutes

9. Remove from the oven and allow the cake to cool completely before icing

10. When it is time to make the icing, place the honey, oil, and cocoa powder into a blender

11. Pulse briefly to mix

12. Now add the coconut milk and blend until smooth. You may have to add a little bit more milk to achieve the consistency you desire

13. Spread icing over your cake evenly

14. Cover the cake with plastic wrap or a cover and place it in the refrigerator until ready to serve

Makes one delicious cake!

~~~~~~~~

 **On the Day of Your Meal**

Here is a crockpot recipe for your side dish that will help keep congestion down on your stovetop. It takes about 6 hours on LOW, but you can cook it on high for 2 to 3 hours. In addition, this dish has lemon flavoring that goes right along with your chicken dish.

Put your sweet potatoes in to cook ahead of time—before you want to construct your casserole. They need to cook about 1 hour, then have time to cool so you can handle them.

Broccoli with Almonds

I am so thankful my family likes broccoli because there are so many different ways you can fix it. It works well in the slow cooker and offers many flavor combinations.

This one is easy to prepare and is packed full of lemon and garlic flavors. Try this alongside your favorite entrée that is cooking in your other big slow cooker!

Ingredients:

- 8 heads of broccoli—florets only

- 2 cups sliced almonds

- 12 garlic cloves, peeled and left whole

- 3 tablespoons olive oil or coconut oil

- ½ cup lemon juice or juice of 4 lemons

- 1 teaspoon salt

- 1 teaspoon black pepper

Directions:

1. Turn your slow cooker on HIGH while you get your ingredients ready

2. Remove the florets from the broccoli stems and place in the slow cooker

3. Sprinkle the almonds over the broccoli

4. Now add the garlic cloves

5. In a small bowl, combine the oil, lemon juice, salt and pepper and mix

6. Drizzle over the broccoli

7. Place the lid on your slow cooker and turn the temperature down to LOW

8. Cook for 5 to 6 hours or until the broccoli is done the way you like it

Makes 6 to 8 servings

~~~~~~~~

Citrus Chicken

This dish requires that you marinade the breast pieces for an hour before cooking so be sure to consider this time element in your preparations.

Ingredients:

- 2 limes – juiced and zested

- 2 lemons – juiced and zested

- 3 tablespoons extra virgin olive oil

- 1 teaspoon black pepper

- 1 teaspoon sea salt

- 8 boneless, skinless chicken breast - pounded to even thickness

- 3 tablespoons coconut oil

- 8 slices aged cheddar cheese (optional—for those who enjoy dairy occasionally)

Directions:

1. Using a container with a lid that will hold all the chicken breasts, add the juice and zest from the limes and lemon, the oil, pepper, and salt

2. Add the chicken breasts that have been pounded

3. Cover with the lid and shake to distribute the marinade over the breast pieces

4. Place the container in the refrigerator for one hour to marinade

5. Taking a large skillet, heat the coconut oil over medium-high heat

6. Remove each chicken breast from the marinade and place in the pan (depending upon the size of your pan, you may have to cook in batches)

7. Cook each chicken breast for 5 minutes on each side, making sure they are completely cooked through

8. For the last couple of minutes on the second side, place a slice of cheddar cheese, if desired, and allow to melt

9. Remove from the pan and place on a serving dish

Makes 8 servings

~~~~~~~~

Sweet Potato Casserole

With this recipe, you cook the sweet potatoes ahead of time – about 1 hour – so allow this time into the preparation of your recipe.

Ingredients:

- 6 large sweet potatoes

- ½ cup butter, melted

- ¼ cup raw honey

- 2 teaspoons pure vanilla extract

- ¼ teaspoon sea salt

- 3 large eggs, beaten

- ½ cup full fat coconut milk

Topping:

- 2 tablespoons coconut flour

- 1 cup almond flour

- 1/8 teaspoon sea salt

- 1 cup pecans, chopped

- 4 tablespoons butter, melted

- 2 tablespoons raw honey

Directions:

1. Preheat your oven to 400 degrees F

2. On a foil-lined cookie sheet, place the sweet potatoes

3. Put them in your preheated oven and bake for 1 hour

4. Remove from the oven and allow to cool. Turn off your oven

5. Once cooled, remove the skins and place the potatoes in a large mixing bowl

6. Preheat your oven to 375 degrees F

7. Prepare a large rectangular baking dish by lightly greasing it with coconut oil

8. Mash the potatoes

9. Now add the melted butter, honey, vanilla, salt, eggs, and milk

10. Mix thoroughly by hand or a hand mixer

11. Pour the potato mixture into your baking dish and spread out evenly in the dish

12. In a small mixing bowl, add the coconut flour, almond flour, salt and pecans and mix thoroughly

13. Using a small microwavable dish, melt the butter and honey until a smooth consistency is achieved

14. Add the butter/honey combination to the dry ingredients and mix

15. Now sprinkle this topping evenly over the potatoes

16. Place your baking dish into your preheated oven and cook for 20 to 25 minutes or until the top is golden brown

Makes 8-10 servings

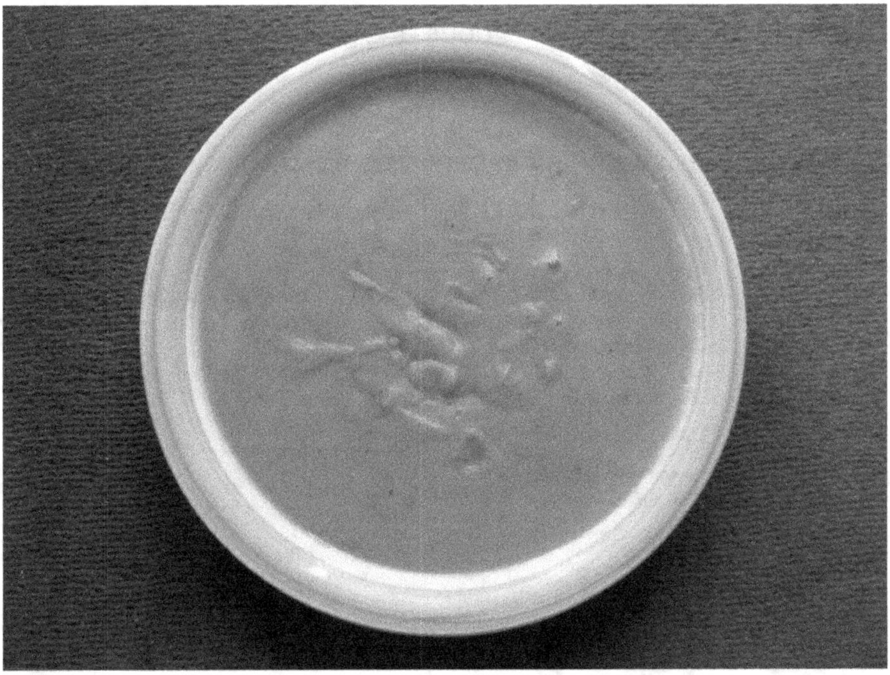

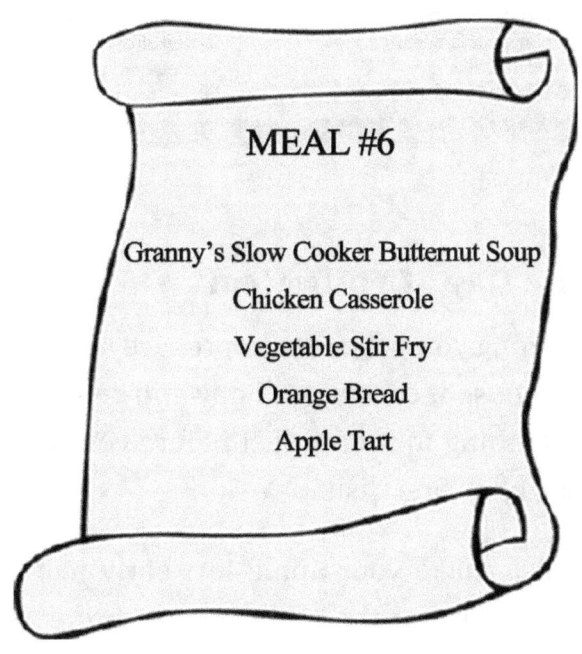

MEAL #6

Granny's Slow Cooker Butternut Soup

Chicken Casserole

Vegetable Stir Fry

Orange Bread

Apple Tart

Main Grocery Items (Foods like salt, pepper, staples and normal pantry items are not included)

Recipe ingredients have been **totaled** so you can see how much you will need for the entire meal (8 servings).

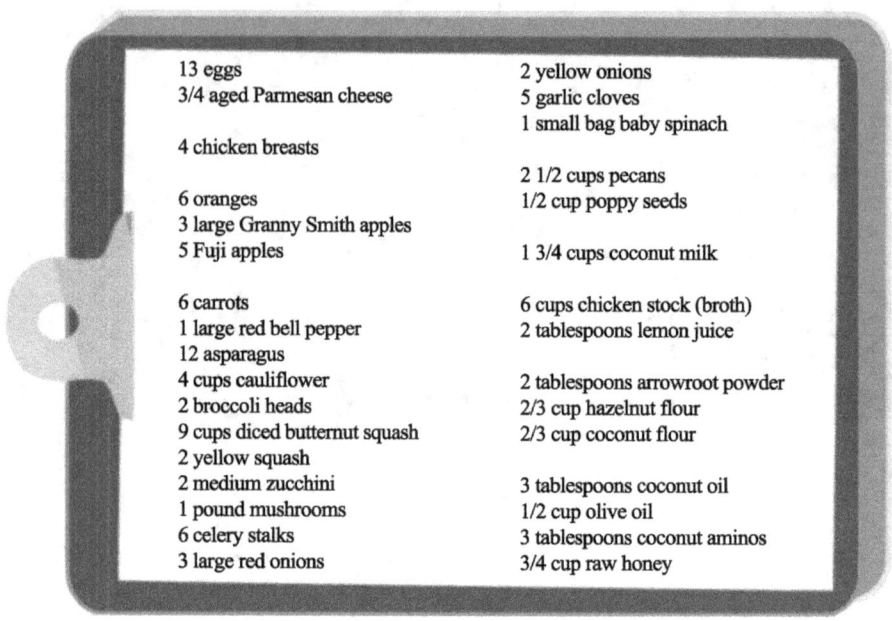

13 eggs
3/4 aged Parmesan cheese

4 chicken breasts

6 oranges
3 large Granny Smith apples
5 Fuji apples

6 carrots
1 large red bell pepper
12 asparagus
4 cups cauliflower
2 broccoli heads
9 cups diced butternut squash
2 yellow squash
2 medium zucchini
1 pound mushrooms
6 celery stalks
3 large red onions

2 yellow onions
5 garlic cloves
1 small bag baby spinach

2 1/2 cups pecans
1/2 cup poppy seeds

1 3/4 cups coconut milk

6 cups chicken stock (broth)
2 tablespoons lemon juice

2 tablespoons arrowroot powder
2/3 cup hazelnut flour
2/3 cup coconut flour

3 tablespoons coconut oil
1/2 cup olive oil
3 tablespoons coconut aminos
3/4 cup raw honey

 **On the Day of Your Meal**

In the morning you will want to prepare the butternut soup for your crockpot so it can cook all day and you will not have to do much of anything to it until just before you want to serve it as your appetizer or first dish.

You can also make your apple tart early in the day, after you put the soup on, or the night before. Either way, all you have to do is warm it up before serving.

Granny's Slow Cooker Butternut Soup

Butternut squash is one of the softer skinned winter squashes so it is easier to cut and peel than several of the other squashes. When the sweetness of the butternut squash meets the tartness of the Granny Smith apples in this soup, an explosion of deliciousness fills your mouth.

Ingredients:

- 3 tablespoons coconut oil

- 3 large red onions (for color. You can use any kind you want)

- 9 cups of diced butternut squash – peeled, seeded and cut into cubes

- 6 celery stalks, cut into slices

- 3 large Granny Smith apples, peeled, cored and chopped

- 6 cups natural chicken broth

- 2 tablespoons kosher or sea salt

- 1 tablespoon coarse black pepper

- ½ teaspoon nutmeg

- ½ teaspoon cinnamon

- ¾ teaspoon cayenne pepper

Directions:

1. Turn your slow cooker on HIGH while you get your ingredients ready

2. On the stovetop, use a large saucepan and melt the coconut oil

3. Place the onions, squash, and celery into the pan and cook until vegetables begin to soften – approximately 10 to 15 minutes.

4. Transfer the vegetables to your slow cooker

5. To the slow cooker, add the chopped apples, chicken broth, salt, pepper, nutmeg, cinnamon, and cayenne pepper

6. Cook on HIGH for 7 to 8 hours and LOW for 10 hours

7. Turn the slow cooker down to WARM if your cooker has this setting; otherwise, LOW

8. Using a stick immerse able blender stick, puree the soup

9. Continue until you have the consistency you desire

10. Taste the soup and adjust the seasonings to your liking

Makes 8-10 servings

~~~~~~~~

Apple Tart

Ingredients:

Crust

- 2½ cups pecans

- ¼ teaspoon sea salt

- 1 teaspoon baking soda

- 2 tablespoons butter, melted

Filling

- 2 tablespoons raw honey, heated so it flows easily

- 2 tablespoons lemon juice

- 2 tablespoons arrowroot powder

- 2 tablespoons ground cinnamon

- 5 medium Fuji apples (or your favorite), peeled, cored and thinly sliced

Directions:

1. Preheat your oven to 350 degrees F

2. Using a food processor, place the pecans, salt, and baking soda inside

3. Pulse until the pecans become finely ground

4. Now add in the melted butter and continue pulsing until totally blended

5. Using a 9-inch tart pan, pour the crust out into it and pat it out across the bottom and up the sides of the tart pan, making the sides slightly thicker than the bottom

6. Place the pan on top of a cookie sheet, bake your crust for 15 minutes

7. Remove from the oven and allow to cool while you make your filling

8. In a large microwavable bowl, put the honey and heat for 20 to 30 seconds so it will flow easier

9. Now add the lemon juice, arrowroot, and cinnamon

10. Stir to blend completely

11. Place your apple slices on top of this mixture and stir until the apples are evenly coated

12. Arrange the apple slices in the tart pan to your liking, making sure they are an even thickness

13. Cover the tart pan with foil and return your pan to the oven and bake for 55 to 60 minutes

14. Remove the foil and cover for 10 minutes more

15. Cool completely

Makes 6 to 8 servings

For the bread, you will be making 4 mini loaves of orange muffins. Because your chicken casserole will be cooking in the oven, it would be best to cook these before the casserole. Then they can cool while the casserole is baking.

Orange Bread

Ingredients:

- ½ cup olive oil

- 2/3 cup raw honey, melted but not hot

- 1 tablespoon pure vanilla extract

- 1 teaspoon almond extract

- 10 eggs

- 4 tablespoons orange jest (try to use 2-3 fresh oranges)

- ½ cup orange juice (try to use fresh)

- ½ cup poppy seeds (optional)

- 2/3 cup hazelnut flour

- 2/3 cup coconut flour (not packed)

- ½ teaspoon sea salt

- 1 teaspoon baking soda

Directions:

1. Preheat your oven to 350 degrees F

2. Prepare 4 mini loaf pans or muffin tins by spreading coconut oil or palm shortening along the sides and bottom

3. In a large mixing bowl, place the olive oil, melted honey, vanilla, almond extract, eggs, orange zest, orange juice, and poppy seeds and blend together

4. Allow the mixture to sit for about 10 minutes so the poppy seeds can plump up while you mix together your dry ingredients

5. In a separate bowl, combine the hazelnut flour, coconut flour, sea salt, and baking soda

6. Using a hand mixer, thoroughly combine the dry ingredients, breaking up any lumps in the flours

7. When you are ready, pour the dry ingredients into the wet ingredients and blend well using your hand mixer

8. Evenly divide the batter between the four pans and place in your preheated oven

9. Bake until the center of the loaves is cooked through—about 35 minutes

10. Once they are baked, allow them to cool inside the pans for about 10 to 15 minutes, then place on wire racks to finish cooling

11. Serve with some butter and be sure to refrigerate any leftovers in an airtight container

Makes 4 mini loaves

~~~~~~~~~

Chicken Casserole

Casseroles are so good and versatile. Feel free to add some of your favorite ingredients to this one when you make it. Have fun with it!

Ingredients:

- 2 carrots, sliced

- 4 cups cauliflower, chopped

- 2 cups broccoli crowns

- 1 stick of butter

- 1¾ cups coconut milk

- 1 teaspoon garlic powder

- ¾ cup aged Parmesan cheese (optional)

- ½ teaspoon sea salt

- ½ yellow onion, chopped

- 3 large eggs

- ½ teaspoon black pepper

- 4 chicken breasts, cooked and cubed

Directions:

1. Preheat oven to 375 degrees F

2. Steam the carrots, cauliflower, and broccoli in your microwave or on your stovetop

3. Set aside

4. Heat the butter in a microwave-safe bowl

5. Add in the coconut milk, garlic powder, Parmesan cheese, salt, onion, eggs, and pepper

6. Mix with a fork or whisk until thoroughly blended

7. Mix in the cooked-cubed chicken, steamed carrots, cauliflower, and broccoli and mix thoroughly

8. Pour into a rectangular casserole dish that has been greased with coconut oil

9. Lightly sprinkle with some additional Parmesan cheese on top

10. Bake for 1 hour

11. Now turn the oven on to broil

12. Once heated, place the casserole under the broiler for 7 to 8 minutes until browned to your liking

Makes 8 servings

~~~~~~~~

Vegetable Stir Fry

Ingredients:

- 2 tablespoons coconut oil

- 5 garlic cloves, peeled and minced

- 1 onion, peeled and diced

- 2 yellow squash, diced

- 2 medium zucchini, diced

- 1 pound mushrooms, sliced

- 2 cups shredded carrots

- 1 large red bell pepper, seeded and cut into thin strips

- 12 asparagus spears, cut into 1-inch pieces

- 1 small bag baby spinach leaves

- 1 - 2 tablespoons coconut aminos

-   Sea salt and pepper to taste

Directions:

1. In a large frying pan, heat the coconut oil

2. Add in the garlic and onion and cook until onion pieces are tender

3. Add the squash, zucchini, mushrooms, carrots, bell pepper, and asparagus and cook until tender

4. Add in the spinach and aminos and cook briefly to allow the spinach to wilt

5. Taste and add salt and pepper to your liking

Makes 8 to 10 servings

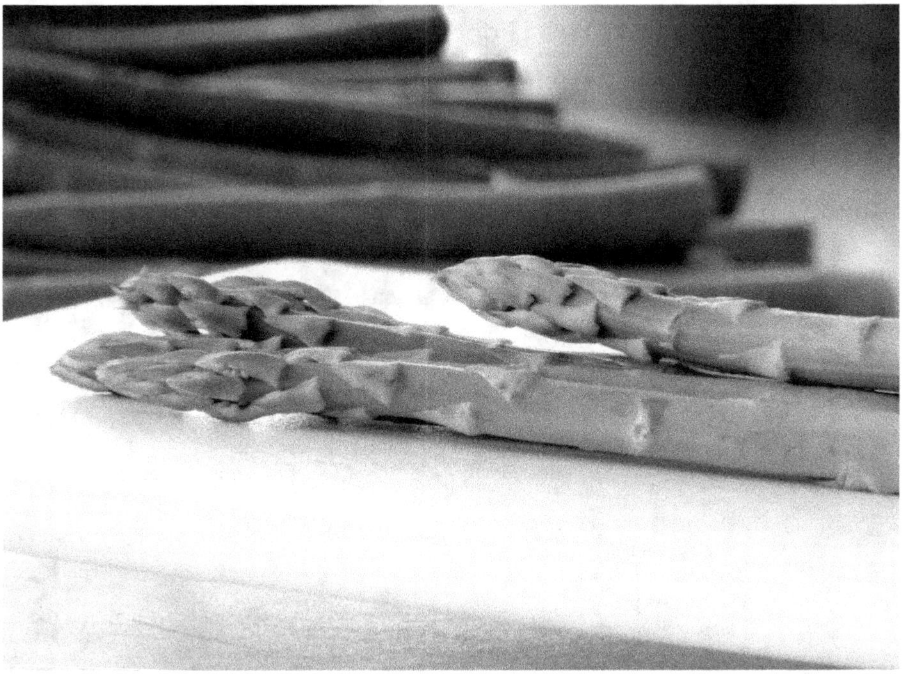

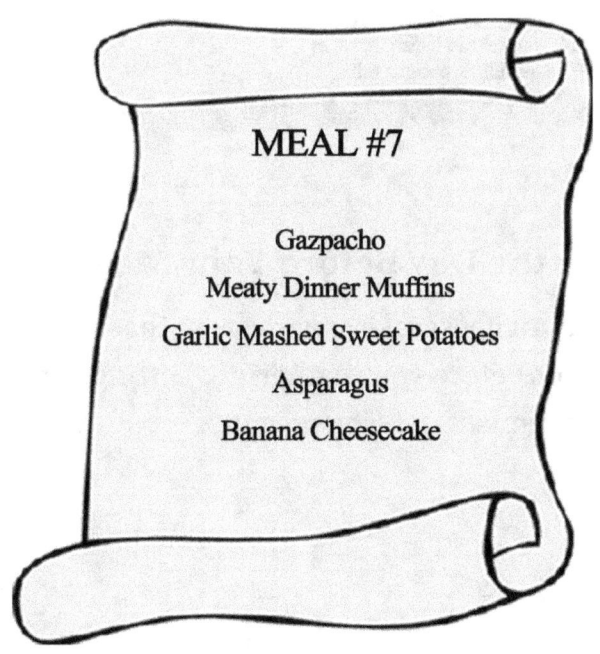

MEAL #7

Gazpacho

Meaty Dinner Muffins

Garlic Mashed Sweet Potatoes

Asparagus

Banana Cheesecake

Main Grocery Items (Foods like salt, pepper, staples and normal pantry items are not included)

Recipe ingredients have been **totaled** so you can see how much you will need for the entire meal (8 servings).

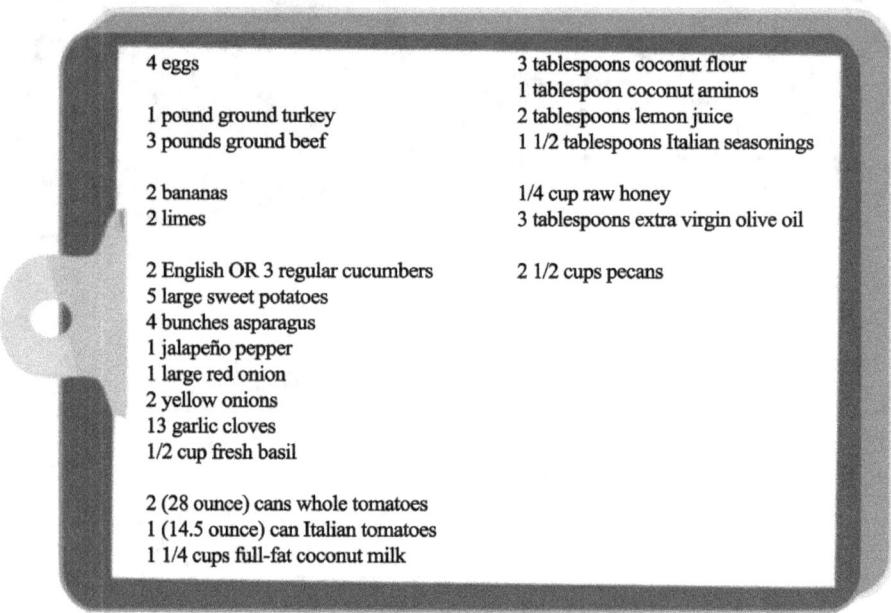

4 eggs

1 pound ground turkey
3 pounds ground beef

2 bananas
2 limes

2 English OR 3 regular cucumbers
5 large sweet potatoes
4 bunches asparagus
1 jalapeño pepper
1 large red onion
2 yellow onions
13 garlic cloves
1/2 cup fresh basil

2 (28 ounce) cans whole tomatoes
1 (14.5 ounce) can Italian tomatoes
1 1/4 cups full-fat coconut milk

3 tablespoons coconut flour
1 tablespoon coconut aminos
2 tablespoons lemon juice
1 1/2 tablespoons Italian seasonings

1/4 cup raw honey
3 tablespoons extra virgin olive oil

2 1/2 cups pecans

**Make the Day Before Your Meal**

The banana cheesecake is a dessert that works best when made the night before your gathering. Letting it firm up in the refrigerator promises delicious results.

Banana Cheesecake

The crust for this cheesecake is the same one used for the apple tart. It works well to put it into a spring form pan to make it easy to cut and serve.

Ingredients:

Crust

- 2½ cups pecans

- ¼ teaspoon sea salt

- 1 teaspoon baking soda

- 2 tablespoons butter, melted

Filling

- 2 eggs (room temperature)

- 2/3 cup full-fat coconut milk

- ¼ cup raw honey

- 1 teaspoon pure vanilla extract

- 2 ripe bananas, peeled

- 3 tablespoons coconut flour

Directions:

1. Preheat your oven to 350 degrees F

2. Using a food processor, place the pecans, salt, and baking soda inside

3. Pulse until the pecans become finely ground

4. Now add in the melted butter and continue pulsing until totally blended

5. Using a 9-inch spring form pan, pour the crust out into it and pat it out across the bottom

6. Place the pan on top of a cookie sheet and bake your crust for 15 minutes

7. Remove from the oven and allow to cool while you make your filling

8. In your blender, put the eggs and process on high for 1 minute. This will help make them fluffy

9. Add the milk, honey, vanilla, bananas, and flour and process until thoroughly blended and smooth

10. Pour the filling into your crust and place in your preheated oven

11. Bake for 30 minutes. The cheesecake is done when it is not wet and giggly in the middle

12. Allow it to cool for 15 to 20 minutes on a wire rack

13. Cover and place in your refrigerator for at least two hours to allow it to set and chill through

Makes 8 servings

~~~~~~~~

Gazpacho

This dish is easy to make and only requires processing in a blender. If your blender isn't very big, you will want to put all the ingredients into a big bowl, then scoop some out and pour into your blender. It's a little bit of trouble, but oh so worth it.

Ingredients:

- 3 garlic cloves, peeled

- 1 large red onion, peeled and cut into smaller pieces

- 2 (28 ounce) cans of organic whole tomatoes

- 2 English cucumbers or 3 regular cucumbers, peeled and diced

- 1 jalapeno pepper with seeds removed

- 1 tablespoon coconut aminos

- 2 tablespoons fresh lime juice

- ½ cup fresh basil leaves

- 1 tablespoon balsamic vinegar

- 1 teaspoon sea salt

- 2 teaspoons coarse black pepper

Directions

1. In a large mixing bowl, place all your ingredients

2. Scoop out some of the mixture and process it in your blender until you achieve the desired consistency

3. Pour the soup out of your blender into a serving bowl or dish

4. Continue processing all the ingredients until you have blended them all

5. This soup is intended to be served cold, but warmed up is delicious as well

Makes 8 to 10 servings

~~~~~~~~

Meaty Dinner Muffins

The fun part about these muffins is they are actually made with ground turkey that are seasoned to taste like sausage and are then combined with ground beef. You can enjoy doing this anytime you find yourself without some sausage but have turkey instead. Just season it and only you will know!

Ingredients:

- 1 (14.5 ounce) can Italian tomatoes, drained

- 2 onions, peeled and quartered

- 1 teaspoon dried sage

- 1 teaspoon dried thyme

- ¼ teaspoon ground nutmeg

- ½ teaspoon onion powder

- 1 teaspoon ground pepper

- 1 pound ground turkey

- 3 pounds ground beef

- 2 eggs

- 2 teaspoons garlic powder

- 1½ tablespoons Italian seasonings

- Salt and pepper to taste

Directions:

1. Preheat your oven to 375 degrees F

2. Lightly grease muffin pans with coconut oil

3. Place drained tomatoes in a food processor along with the onion

4. In a small bowl, combine the sage, thyme, nutmeg, onion powder, and pepper together and mix thoroughly

5. In a large separate bowl, mix this seasoning mix into the ground turkey thoroughly to create "sausage"

6. Now add the beef, egg, garlic, seasonings, salt and pepper and the tomato/onion puree in with the ground turkey

7. Fill up the muffin tins about three-fourths of the way full with the meat mixture

8. Place in the preheated oven for 30 - 45 minutes

Serves 8 to 10 people

~~~~~~~~

Garlic Mashed Sweet Potatoes

Ingredients:

- 2 tablespoons extra virgin olive oil

- 5 garlic cloves, peeled and minced

- 1 teaspoon coarse black pepper

- 2 teaspoons sea salt

- 5 large sweet potatoes, peeled and diced

- 1 teaspoon lemon juice

- ½ cup full fat coconut milk

- 1 teaspoon ground cinnamon

- 1/8 teaspoon cayenne pepper

Directions:

1. Preheat your oven to 400 degrees F

2. In a large bowl, place the oil, garlic, pepper, and salt and mix to combine

3. Add the potato dices and coat with the liquid

4. Pour the potatoes out onto a baking sheet that has been treated with coconut oil and spread out evenly

5. Place in your preheated oven and bake for 25 to 30 minutes

6. In a large mixing bowl, pour the lemon juice, coconut milk, cinnamon and pepper

7. Using a hand mixer, blend completely

8. Once the potatoes are done, add them to this liquid and carefully break up the potatoes with the mixer and blend until smooth

Makes 8 to 10 servings

~~~~~~~~

While you are taking the sweet potatoes out of the oven, place the asparagus in so it can cook while you process the potatoes. Just be sure to lower the temperature to 375 degrees F when you do.

Asparagus

Ingredients:

- 3 tablespoons extra virgin olive oil

- 2 tablespoons lemon juice

- 5 garlic cloves, peeled and minced

- 1½ teaspoons sea salt

- 1 teaspoon coarse black pepper

- 1/8 teaspoon cayenne pepper

- 4 bunches fresh asparagus, bottoms trimmed

Directions:

1. Preheat your oven to 375 degrees F

2. In a small bowl, combine the oil, lemon juice, garlic, salt, pepper, and cayenne pepper

3. Mix thoroughly

4. On a baking sheet that has a lip to it, put the asparagus and then pour the liquid over it and toss it evenly

5. Place the baking sheet into your oven and bake for 15 to 20 minutes, turning it halfway through the baking time

Makes 6 to 8 servings

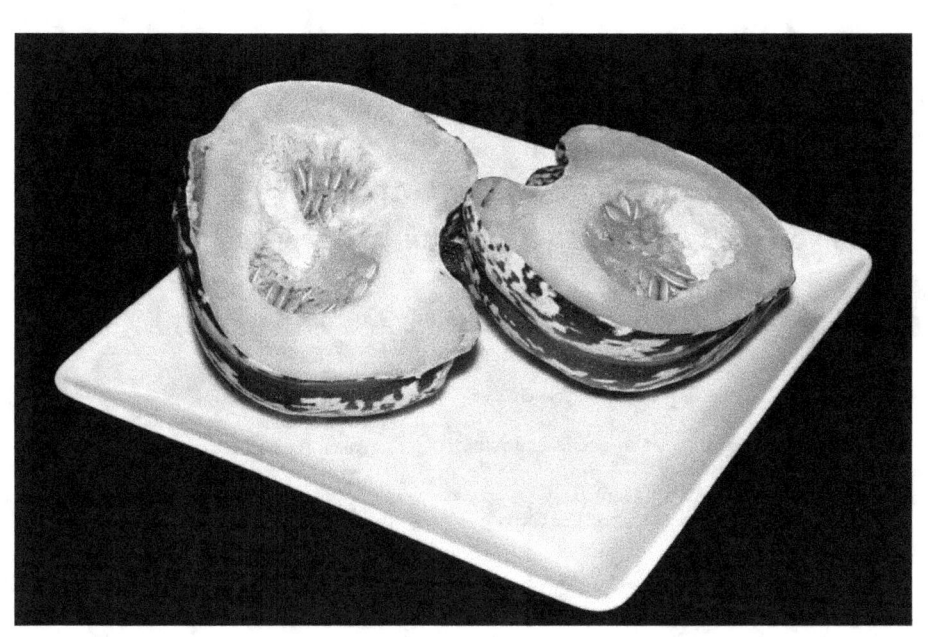

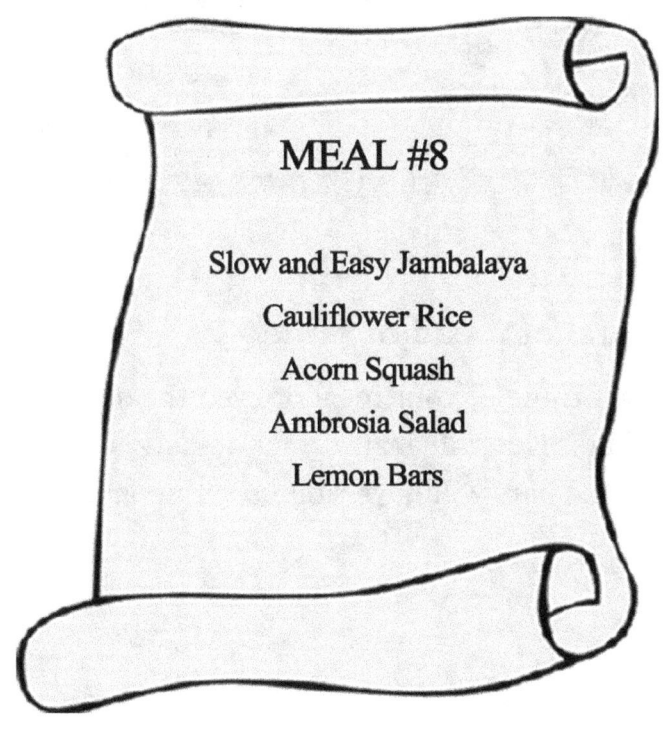

MEAL #8

Slow and Easy Jambalaya

Cauliflower Rice

Acorn Squash

Ambrosia Salad

Lemon Bars

Main Grocery Items (Foods like salt, pepper, staples and normal pantry items are not included)

Recipe ingredients have been **totaled** so you can see how much you will need for the entire meal (8 servings).

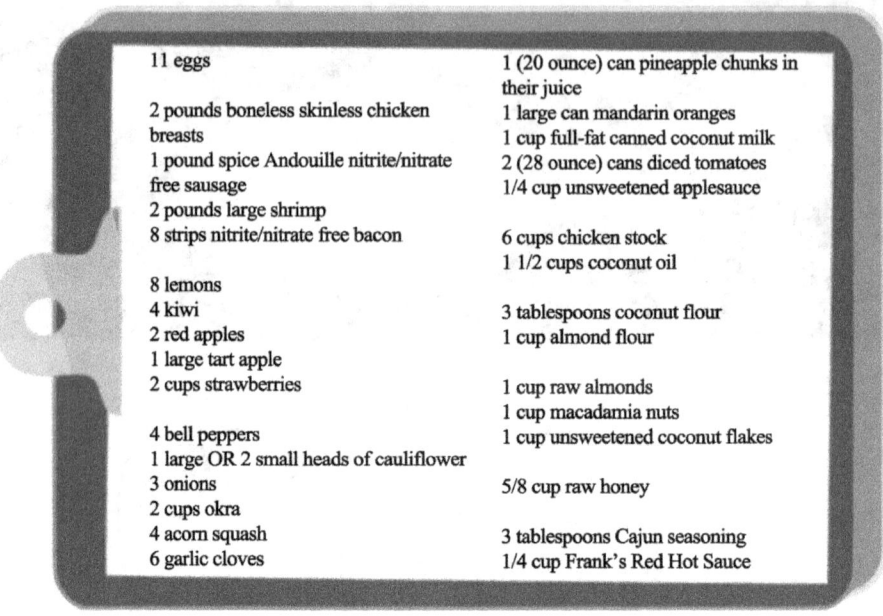

11 eggs	1 (20 ounce) can pineapple chunks in their juice
2 pounds boneless skinless chicken breasts	1 large can mandarin oranges
1 pound spice Andouille nitrite/nitrate free sausage	1 cup full-fat canned coconut milk
2 pounds large shrimp	2 (28 ounce) cans diced tomatoes
8 strips nitrite/nitrate free bacon	1/4 cup unsweetened applesauce
8 lemons	6 cups chicken stock
4 kiwi	1 1/2 cups coconut oil
2 red apples	3 tablespoons coconut flour
1 large tart apple	1 cup almond flour
2 cups strawberries	1 cup raw almonds
4 bell peppers	1 cup macadamia nuts
1 large OR 2 small heads of cauliflower	1 cup unsweetened coconut flakes
3 onions	5/8 cup raw honey
2 cups okra	3 tablespoons Cajun seasoning
4 acorn squash	1/4 cup Frank's Red Hot Sauce
6 garlic cloves	

 ## To Make Ahead of Time

On the morning of your meal or even the day before, make the lemon bars. This will ensure your dessert is ready in plenty of time and the bars will have time to set up and develop their flavor.

Lemon Bars

Ingredients:

Topping

- 6 eggs

- ½ cup raw honey

- Juice from 8 lemons (1 cup)

- ½ cup coconut oil

- ½ - ¾ cup unsweetened coconut flakes for topping

Crust

- 1 cup raw almonds

- 1 cup macadamia nuts

- ¼ cup raw honey

- ½ cup coconut oil, melted

- 2 eggs

Directions:

1. Preheat your oven to 400 degrees F

2. Using a medium saucepan, stir together the eggs, honey, and lemon juice over medium-high heat

3. Now add the coconut oil

4. Continue stirring until the mixture thickens and begins to bubble

5. Remove from heat

6. Pour mixture into a bowl and place in your refrigerator to cool

7. Using a food processor, add the almonds and macadamia nuts

8. Pulse at intervals until you have the nuts in small chunks. Do not process too much or you will have a flour mixture. You want a coarse, chunky texture

9. Into a mixing bowl, place the nut mixture, honey, melted oil, and eggs and mix thoroughly

10. Using coconut oil or olive oil, grease a rectangular pan

11. Spread the mixture into the pan evenly

12. Bake for 15 to 20 minutes until the crust is done

13. Remove from the oven and cool completely

14. Once the crust is cooled, take your lemon mixture out of the refrigerator and spread over the crust

15. If desired, sprinkle shredded coconut over the top and return to the refrigerator

16. Once thoroughly cooled, slice and eat

17. Keep any leftovers sealed in an airtight container in your refrigerator.

~~~~~~~~

On the morning of your meal, make this ambrosia salad so it has time to chill. It will save you time later. You do not have to worry about your apples turning brown either because the pineapple juice will help to preserve their color.

Ambrosia Salad

Ingredients:

- 1 (20 ounce) can pineapple chunks in their own juice

- 4 kiwi - peeled and sliced

- 2 red apples - cut into small chunks (I love Fuji or Honeycrisp)

- 2 cups strawberries, halved or quartered

- 1 large can mandarin oranges -- drained

- 1 cup full-fat canned coconut milk

- ¼ cup raw honey (warmed slightly to make it easier to pour and mix)

- ¼ cup unsweetened shredded coconut

- ¾ teaspoon ground cinnamon

Directions

1. In a large bowl, add the pineapple, kiwi, apples, strawberries, and oranges

2. Mix gently

3. In a smaller bowl, combine the coconut milk and honey to create a smooth consistency

4. Sprinkle the coconut and cinnamon over the fruit

5. Now add the dressing and mix until thoroughly blended

6. Cover and refrigerate until ready to serve

7. Can be placed on a bed of lettuce leaves for a fruit salad dish or served in small dessert bowls

Makes 8 servings

~~~~~~~~

Slow and Easy Jambalaya

Here is a jambalaya recipe that will have your house smelling delicious all day long while it slowly simmers to perfection.

Ingredients:

- 6 cups chicken stock

- 4 bell peppers, chopped

- 2 onions, peeled and chopped

- 4 garlic cloves, diced

- 2 (28 ounce) cans of diced tomatoes—do NOT drain

- 4 bay leaves

- 2 pounds boneless skinless chicken breasts, diced

- 3 tablespoons Cajun seasoning

- ¼ cup Frank's Red Hot sauce or hot sauce of your choice

- 1 pound spicy Andouille nitrite/nitrate-free sausage (optional)

- 2 pounds large shrimp, raw and deveined

- 2 cups okra, sliced

Directions:

1. Turn your slow cooker on HIGH while you get your ingredients ready

2. Pour the chicken stock, bell peppers, onion, garlic, diced tomatoes with juice, bay leaves, chicken, Cajun seasoning, and hot sauce into your slow cooker

3. Now turn your slow cooker down to LOW and cook for 6 hours

4. Thirty minutes before the jambalaya is due to be finished, gently toss in the sausage, raw shrimp and okra

99

5. Mix ingredients together and continue cooking until the shrimp is done – approximately 30 minutes to one hour

6. Serve over cauliflower rice (recipe below)

Makes 8 to 10 servings

If you only happen to have 1 large crockpot, you may need to either borrow one or cook your jambalaya in a large soup pot on your stovetop. Alternatively, let the jambalaya cook in your crockpot and cook the apple cinnamon bread in your oven on 350 degrees for 35 to 40 minutes. Have two large crockpots like me? No problem!

Apple Cinnamon Bread

Ingredients:

- 3 eggs (room temperature)

- ¼ cup coconut oil, melted

- 2 tablespoons raw honey or pure maple syrup

- ¼ cup unsweetened applesauce

- 3 tablespoons coconut flour

- 1 cup almond flour

- 1 heaping tablespoon cinnamon

- ½ teaspoon baking soda

- ½ teaspoon sea salt

- 1 large, tart apple, peeled, cored and diced

Directions:

1. Turn on your slow cooker to HIGH while you get your ingredients ready

2. Spray or apply coconut oil to the sides and bottom of your loaf pan

3. In a blender, put the eggs, coconut oil, honey, and apple sauce

4. Allow the blender to run on low or medium while you mix up the dry ingredients in a bowl

5. Place the apple pieces in the dry ingredients and coat them with the flour, etc.

6. Pour the ingredients in the blender into the dry ingredients and mix thoroughly

7. Pour the batter into the loaf pan

8. Place the lid on your slow cooker, using a couple of toothpicks to prop it up to reduce any condensation

9. Cook on HIGH for 2 hours

10. Using a toothpick, check for doneness

11. Remove from the slow cooker and place the pan on a cooling rack for 15 minutes

12. Using a knife, scrape the sides loose and gently invert the bread pan so the loaf is on the cooling rack

13. Allow to cool completely

14. Slice and butter if desired

Makes 1 loaf

With the bread safely in the crockpot, now would be a good time to cook the squash halves in the oven. This will allow them to cook and cool off so you can scoop them out without getting burned.

Acorn Squash

Ingredients

- 4 acorn squash, cut in half

- 8 strips of bacon, diced

- 2 tablespoons ground cinnamon

- 4 tablespoons butter

- 1 teaspoon sea salt

Directions

1. Preheat your oven to 400 degrees F

2. Line a cookie sheet with foil and then put each acorn half face down on the foil for baking

3. Place the cookie sheet into your preheated oven and cook for 30 minutes. The squash will be done when you can easily insert a knife through the skin from the outside

4. While the squash is in the oven, place a skillet on your stovetop over medium to high heat and cook the bacon pieces

5. Turn off the heat and remove the bacon pieces and allow them to drain

6. In a medium mixing bowl, add 1 tablespoon of bacon drippings from the skillet

7. Add the bacon pieces to the bowl

8. Once the squash is cool enough to handle, scoop out the shells and add the flesh to the bowl

9. Add the cinnamon, butter, and salt and blend thoroughly to create a smooth consistency

10. Evenly divide the mixture into the acorn squash shells, lightly sprinkle with cinnamon and serve

Makes 8 servings

~~~~~~~~

Once you put the shrimp and okra into your slow cooker, that is the time to make the cauliflower rice so it will be all ready when it is time to serve your meal.

Cauliflower Rice

Ingredients:

- 2 tablespoons coconut oil

- 1 onion, peeled and finely diced

- 2 garlic cloves, peeled and minced

- 1 large or 2 small heads of cauliflower

- 3 tablespoons butter

- 1½ teaspoons sea salt

- Favorite seasonings

Directions

1. Clean the cauliflower and break it up into pieces that will fit inside your food processor

2. Pulse until the cauliflower has a "rice" consistency

3. On your stovetop, place a large skillet over medium heat with the coconut oil

4. Once the oil is heated, add the onion pieces and garlic to the skillet

5. Sauté until the onion becomes tender

6. Now add the cauliflower rice to the saucepan

7. Mix together with the onion and garlic, then cover

8. Cook for approximately 8 to 10 minutes

9. Remove the cover and add the butter and any special seasoning you would like for the cauliflower to have once it is under the jambalaya

10. Stir the ingredients together

11. Now the rice is ready

Makes 10 to 12 servings

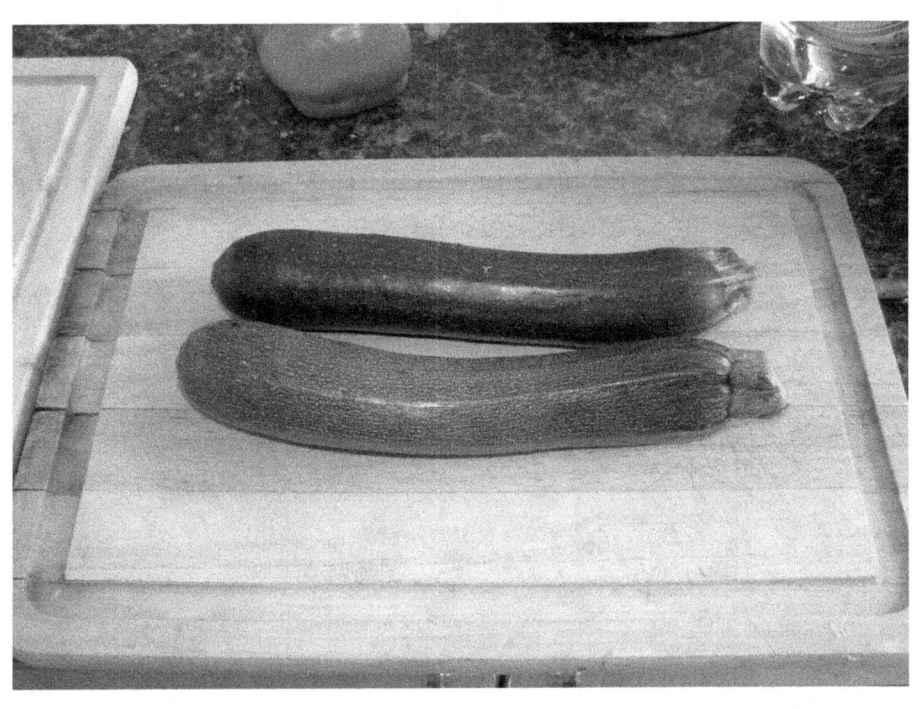

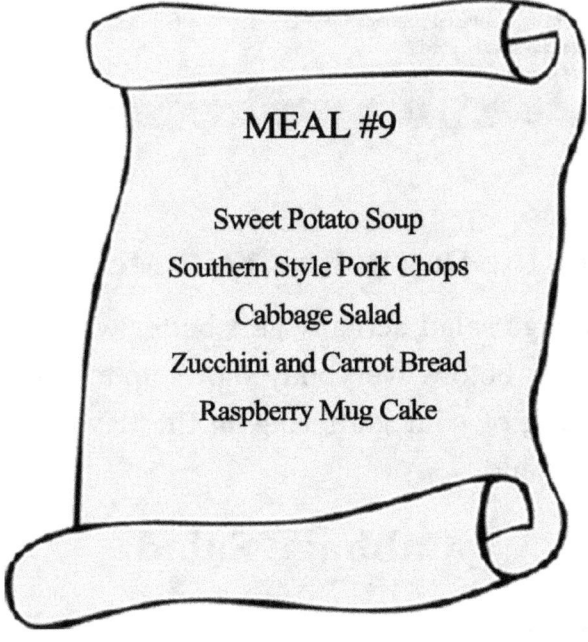

MEAL #9

Sweet Potato Soup

Southern Style Pork Chops

Cabbage Salad

Zucchini and Carrot Bread

Raspberry Mug Cake

Main Grocery Items (Foods like salt, pepper, staples and normal pantry items are not included)

Recipe ingredients have been **totaled** so you can see how much you will need for the entire meal (8 servings).

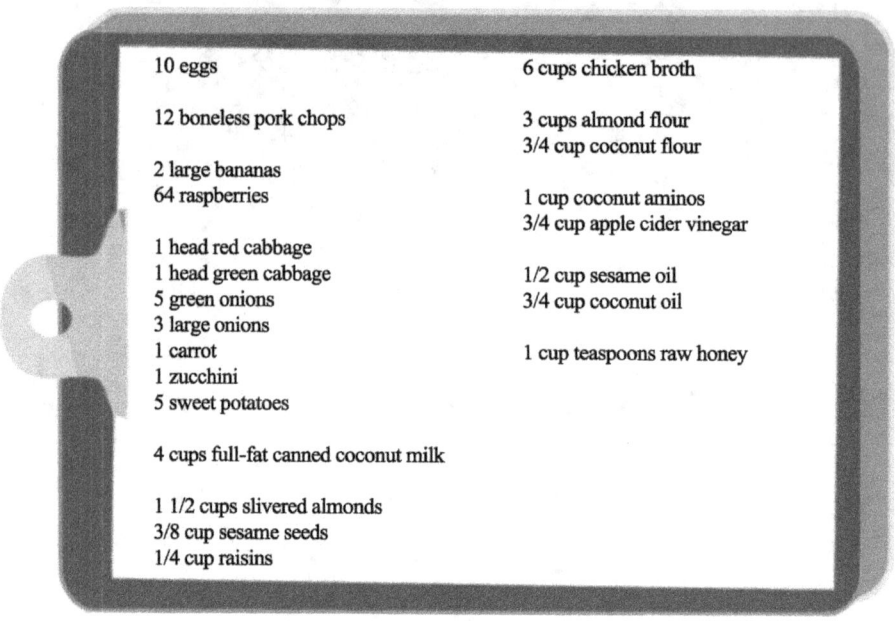

10 eggs	6 cups chicken broth
12 boneless pork chops	3 cups almond flour
	3/4 cup coconut flour
2 large bananas	
64 raspberries	1 cup coconut aminos
	3/4 cup apple cider vinegar
1 head red cabbage	
1 head green cabbage	1/2 cup sesame oil
5 green onions	3/4 cup coconut oil
3 large onions	
1 carrot	1 cup teaspoons raw honey
1 zucchini	
5 sweet potatoes	
4 cups full-fat canned coconut milk	
1 1/2 cups slivered almonds	
3/8 cup sesame seeds	
1/4 cup raisins	

**Make the Day Before Your Meal**

This cabbage salad actually gets better with time so try to make it the day before everybody shows up to eat or very early in the morning of your gathering so the flavors have time to develop and blend.

Cabbage Salad

Ingredients:

- 1 head of red cabbage, shredded

- 1 head of green cabbage, shredded

- 1½ cups slivered almonds

- 3/8 cup roasted sesame seeds

- 5 green onions, chopped

- 2 teaspoons coarse black pepper

- 1 cup coconut aminos (in place of soy sauce)

- ¾ cup apple cider vinegar

- ½ cup sesame oil

- 2 teaspoons raw honey

Directions:

1. In a large mixing bowl, combine the red and green cabbages, almonds, sesame seeds, onions, and pepper and toss together

2. In a small to medium bowl, combine the aminos, cider vinegar, oil, and honey and mix thoroughly

3. Pour the dressing over the cabbage and mix until the cabbage is thoroughly coated

4. Taste and adjust the seasoning by adding salt, more pepper, etc.

5. Cover and place in the refrigerator to chill completely

Makes 8-10 servings

**Early on the Day of Your Meal**

You will want to cook your sweet potatoes early enough in the day so they have time to completely cool. This will allow you to peel them easily and cube them to go into your soup later.

For the next step, get out your crockpot so you can make some bread for your meal. It takes about two hours in the crockpot, plus the time it takes you to mix things up.

Zucchini and Carrot Bread

Ingredients:

- 2 large eggs (room temperature)

- ¼ cup raw honey or pure maple syrup

- ¼ cup coconut oil

- 1 teaspoon of pure vanilla extract

- 1 tablespoon of coconut flour

- 2 cups almond flour

- 1 tablespoon ground cinnamon

- ½ teaspoon of baking soda

- ½ teaspoon of sea salt

- 1 carrot, grated (1/2 cup)

- 1 zucchini, grated (3/4 cup)

- ¼ cup raisins

Directions:

1. Turn on your slow cooker to HIGH while you get your ingredients ready

2. Spray or apply coconut oil to the sides and bottom of your loaf pan

3. In a blender, put the eggs, honey, oil, and vanilla

4. Allow the blender to run on low or medium while you mix up the dry ingredients in a bowl

5. Add the wet ingredients into the dry ingredients and mix thoroughly

6. Stir in the carrot, zucchini, and raisins

7. Pour the batter into the loaf pan

8. Place the lid on your slow cooker, using a couple of toothpicks to prop it up to reduce any condensation

9. Cook on HIGH for 2 hours

10. Using a toothpick, check for doneness

11. Remove from the slow cooker and place the pan on a cooling rack for 15 minutes

12. Using a knife, scrape the sides loose and gently invert the bread pan so the loaf is on the cooling rack

13. Allow to cool completely

14. Slice and butter if desired

Makes 1 loaf

~~~~~~~~~

Sweet Potato Soup

Ingredients:

- 3 tablespoons coconut flour

- 3 tablespoons coconut oil

- 4 cups chicken broth

- 5 medium sweet potatoes, cooked and cubed

- 1 teaspoon ground ginger

- ½ teaspoon ground cinnamon

- ½ teaspoon ground nutmeg

- 3 cups canned coconut milk

- Salt and pepper to taste

Directions:

1. In a saucepan over medium-low heat, cook the coconut flour and coconut oil, stirring constantly until the mixture turns a light caramel color

2. Add the chicken broth and bring it to a boil

3. Turn the heat down to low and stir in the sweet potatoes, ginger, cinnamon, and nutmeg

4. Cook on low for 5 more minutes and blend thoroughly

5. Remove from the pot and place the mixture into a blender. (Depending upon the size of your blender, you may have to do this in a couple of batches)

6. Blend the soup until it is a smooth consistency

7. Now return to the saucepan

8. Add the coconut milk and gently reheat the soup

9. Season with salt and pepper and serve

Makes 8 servings

~~~~~~~~

Southern Style Pork Chops

Depending upon the size of your dinner party, you may have to cook the pork chops in batches. However, once they are cooked, we will put them all back together in one dish so they are all finished at the same time.

Ingredients:

- 4 tablespoons coconut flour

- 1 cup almond flour or meal

- 2 tablespoons onion powder

- 2 tablespoons garlic powder

- ½ teaspoon paprika

- 1 tablespoon sea salt

- 2 teaspoons coarse black pepper

- ¾ teaspoon cayenne pepper

- ¼ cup coconut oil for frying

- 12 (4-6 ounce) boneless pork chops

- 3 large onions, peeled and sliced—pop out into rings

- 2 cups chicken broth

- 1 cup full fat coconut milk

Directions:

1. In a wide mixing bowl, combine the coconut flour, almond flour, onion powder, garlic powder, paprika, salt, pepper, and cayenne pepper and stir until well blended

2. Rinse each pork chop under cold water and then pat dry

3. Place a large skillet with a lid (one that will accommodate all your cooked pork chops later) on your stovetop and put the coconut oil in it to heat up

4. Dip each pork chop into the flour mixture to coat each side (Do not discard any remaining mixture because you will be using it later)

5. Place pork chops into the hot oil and cook for 4 to 5 minutes on each side

6. Cook several batches if necessary

7. Once the pork chops are finished cooking and removed from your pan, place your onion rings into the skillet for about 10 to 15 minutes. This should cause them to brown nicely

8. Turn your stovetop setting down to low heat now

9. When the onions are browned, pour whatever remaining flour mixture you had left over the browned onions

10. Now add in the chicken broth and stir together to completely blend in the flour

11. Allow this to cook over low heat for approximately 7 to 8 minutes. This should thicken your sauce some

12. Once slightly thickened, add in your coconut milk

13. At this point, place all the cooked pork chops back into your pan and cover

14. Allow them to continue to cook for an additional 8 to 10 minutes

15. Serve hot

Makes 12 servings

~~~~~~~~

Mug cakes are fun and very versatile. You can make them individually and cook them in a microwave for about two minutes or bake them in your oven. If speed is what you want, go for the microwave but if you have time, I like the consistency better from the oven.

Additionally, you can make this fun by letting your guests and family make their own. You provide the ingredients, tell them how to make them, then either microwave each one (which means the first ones are finished eating while the rest are waiting to cook theirs) or put all of them in the oven to bake together (my preference).

Raspberry Mug Cake

Ingredients:

- 3 tablespoons mashed ripe banana (about a 1-inch slice)

- 8 fresh raspberries

- 1 egg, beaten

- 2 teaspoons raw honey

- 1 teaspoon pure vanilla extract

- 1½ tablespoons coconut flour

- 1/8 teaspoon sea salt

- ½ teaspoon baking powder

Directions:

1. Preheat your oven to 350 degree F if you are going to bake it

2. In a ramekin or coffee mug, put the banana slice and raspberries and smash them with a fork

3. Now add the egg, honey, and vanilla and mix until the egg is beaten

4. Add in the flour, salt, and baking powder, making sure to blend well so you do not get a mouthful of baking powder later

5. **Microwave:** Place the mug inside the microwave and process on high for 2 minutes

6. **Oven:** Place the mug or ramekin on a baking sheet and bake for 30 minutes

7. Remove your cake from the oven carefully and enjoy when the cake has had some time to cool and set up

Makes 1 serving

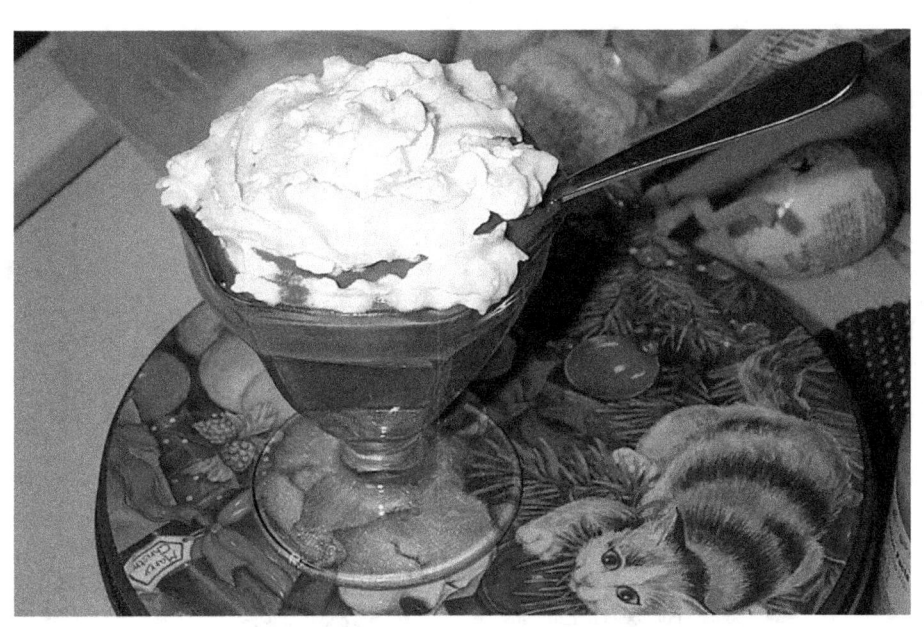

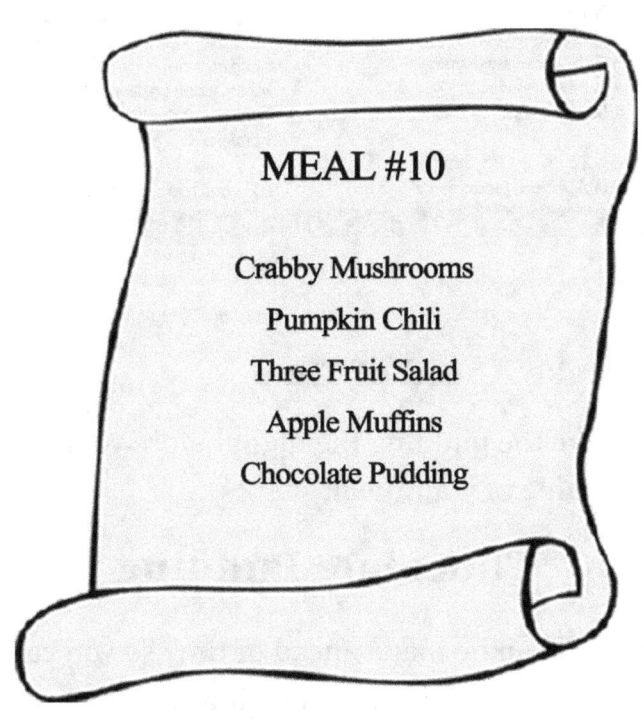

MEAL #10

Crabby Mushrooms

Pumpkin Chili

Three Fruit Salad

Apple Muffins

Chocolate Pudding

Main Grocery Items (Foods like salt, pepper, staples and normal pantry items are not included)

Recipe ingredients have been **totaled** so you can see how much you will need for the entire meal (8 servings).

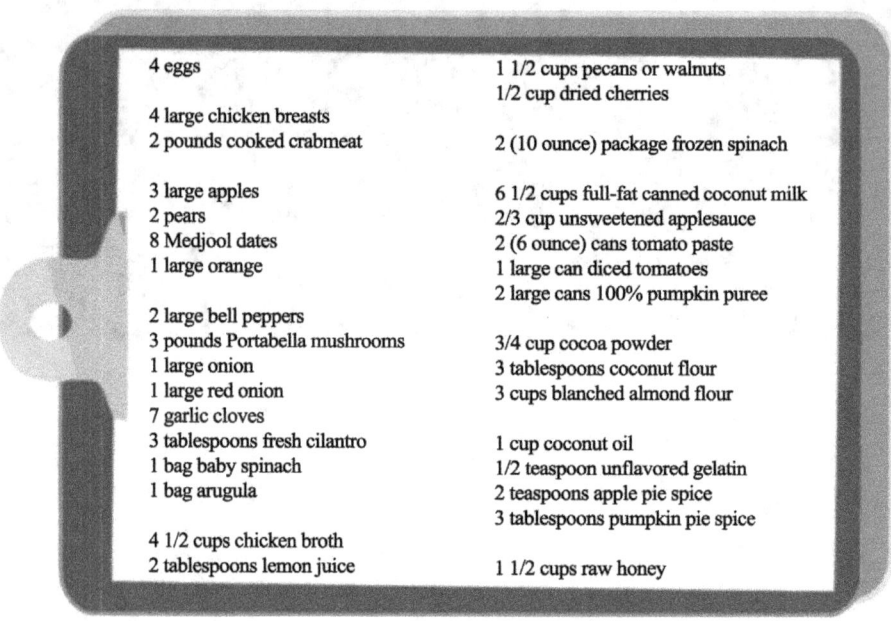

4 eggs	1 1/2 cups pecans or walnuts
	1/2 cup dried cherries
4 large chicken breasts	
2 pounds cooked crabmeat	2 (10 ounce) package frozen spinach
3 large apples	6 1/2 cups full-fat canned coconut milk
2 pears	2/3 cup unsweetened applesauce
8 Medjool dates	2 (6 ounce) cans tomato paste
1 large orange	1 large can diced tomatoes
	2 large cans 100% pumpkin puree
2 large bell peppers	
3 pounds Portabella mushrooms	3/4 cup cocoa powder
1 large onion	3 tablespoons coconut flour
1 large red onion	3 cups blanched almond flour
7 garlic cloves	
3 tablespoons fresh cilantro	1 cup coconut oil
1 bag baby spinach	1/2 teaspoon unflavored gelatin
1 bag arugula	2 teaspoons apple pie spice
	3 tablespoons pumpkin pie spice
4 1/2 cups chicken broth	
2 tablespoons lemon juice	1 1/2 cups raw honey

**To Make Ahead of Time**

Either make the pudding the night before your gathering or early the morning of your meal.

Chocolate Pudding

This dessert can be made ahead of time so you can sit down with your guests or family and enjoy it right along with them

Ingredients:

- ¾ cup arrowroot

- 1 teaspoon salt

- ¾ cup unsweetened cocoa powder

- 6 cups full-fat canned coconut milk (about 4)

- 1½ cups raw honey

- 1½ tablespoons pure vanilla extract

Directions:

1. In a large saucepan on your stovetop, use a whisk to blend the arrowroot, salt, and cocoa powder

2. Pour in 1 cup of milk and blend

3. Using a medium heat setting, stir this mixture until it begins to dissolve and become smooth

4. Add the honey and the rest of the coconut milk and continue to heat

5. Continue to heat until the pudding thickens

6. When thickness is achieved, remove the saucepan from the heat

7. Add the vanilla and stir completely

8. Dish the pudding into serving dishes and chill for at least 3 hours before serving

Makes 8 to 10 servings

 **On the Day of Your Meal**

Prepare the fruit for your salad and place it in an airtight container in the refrigerator until just before you want to serve it. Then toss in with the greens and nuts and top with a favorite dressing.

Three Fruit Salad

Ingredients:

- 2 red apples, cored and diced (Fuji or Gala work well)

- 2 pears, cored and diced

- ½ cup dried cherries

- ½ cup orange juice (1 large orange)

- 1 bag baby spinach leaves

- 1 bag arugula

- ½ cup walnuts or pecans, chopped

- 1 teaspoon ground cinnamon

Directions:

1. In a medium bowl, place the apple pieces, pears, cherries, and orange juice

2. Toss to coat the fruit and allow them to sit for 1/2 hour to rehydrate the cherries some

3. In a large salad bowl, combine the spinach and arugula, nuts and add the cherries and apple pieces and toss

4. Sprinkle on the ground cinnamon

5. Serve and apply your favorite dressing

Makes 8 servings

~~~~~~~~

Apple Muffins

Ingredients:

- 2/3 cup unsweetened applesauce

- 4 eggs

- ½ cup full-fat coconut milk

- ½ cup coconut oil, melted

- 8 Medjool dates, pitted

- ½ tablespoon vanilla extract

- 3 tablespoons coconut flour

- 3 cups blanched almond flour

- ½ teaspoon unflavored gelatin

- 1 teaspoon baking soda

- ½ teaspoon sea salt

- 2 teaspoons apple pie spice

- 1 tablespoon ground cinnamon

- 1 large apple, finely chopped or shredded

- 1 cup chopped pecans or walnuts (optional)

Directions:

1. Preheat your oven to 350 degrees F

2. Lightly grease 24 muffin tins with coconut oil

3. In your food processor, add the applesauce, eggs, milk, oil and dates

4. Process until the dates are completely broken up and blended in with the other ingredients

5. Open up the processor and add the vanilla, flours, gelatin, soda, salt, pie spice, and cinnamon and blend until thoroughly blended throughout

6. Empty the content out of the processor into a large bowl

7. Fold in the apple pieces

8. Evenly divide the batter into your muffin tins

9. Place in your preheated oven and bake for approximately 30 minutes. Make sure the centers are cooked through

10. Remove from your oven, allow them to remain in the tins for 10 to 15 minutes, then serve warm

Makes 24 muffins

~~~~~~~~

While your muffins are cooking in the oven, prepare the ingredients for your mushroom appetizers.

Crabby Mushrooms

Ingredients:

- 2 (10 ounce) packages frozen spinach, thawed

- 3 pounds Portabella mushrooms

- 2 – 3 tablespoons coconut oil

- 1 large onion, chopped

- 4 garlic cloves, minced

- ½ cup chicken broth

- 2 tablespoons lemon juice

- 1 teaspoon dried basil

- 1/2 teaspoon ground ginger

- 1 teaspoon dried oregano

- 2 pounds cooked crabmeat

Directions:

1. Preheat your oven to 425 degrees F

2. Begin by squeezing as much of the excess liquid from your thawed spinach as you can

3. Remove the stems and some of the inside flesh of the mushroom with a spoon

4. Chop some of the stems to make enough for 3 cups

5. In a large skillet, heat up the coconut oil over medium heat

6. Once heated, put the chopped mushroom stems, onion, garlic, broth, and lemon juice into the pan

7. Cook until the onion is tender

8. Now add the spinach and cook until the liquid is evaporated

9. Stir in the basil, ginger and oregano into the spinach

10. Now add the crabmeat and mix gently

11. Spoon the crab mixture into the mushroom tops

12. Place the stuffed mushroom tops onto a lightly greased baking dish

13. Bake for 10 to 15 minutes until the mushrooms are tender

14. Remove from the oven and serve

If you can't find Portabella mushrooms, just get some big button mushrooms and stuff them.

Makes 8 servings

Just before you put the mushrooms into the oven, toss the fruit you prepared earlier with the greens and nuts. Once you put the mushrooms into the oven to bake, you can put your chili together.

Pumpkin Chili

Ingredients:

- 3 tablespoons coconut oil

- 2 large bell peppers (any color), seeded and chopped

- 3 garlic cloves, peeled and minced

- 1 large red onion, peeled and chopped

- 4 cups chicken broth

- 2 (6 ounce) cans tomato paste

- 1 large can diced tomatoes, undrained

- 4 large chicken breasts cut into cubes

- 3 tablespoons pumpkin pie spice

- 2 teaspoons ground coriander

- 3 tablespoons chili powder

- 2 teaspoons ground cinnamon

- 1 teaspoon sea salt

- 2 large cans 100% pumpkin puree

- 3 tablespoons fresh cilantro, chopped

Directions:

1. In a large saucepan or Dutch oven on top of your stove, place the coconut oil and heat it

2. Add the peppers, garlic, and onion and cook until tender

3. Slowly add the chicken broth, tomato paste and diced tomatoes and stir

4. Allow this to heat up for 3 to 4 minutes

5. Add the chicken pieces and cook for 20 to 25 minutes

6. Now add the pie spice, coriander, chili powder, cinnamon and salt

7. Stir thoroughly

8. Add the pumpkin and blend completely

9. Allow the chili to heat through completely

10. Serve when ready to eat and sprinkle the top of each bowl of chili with fresh cilantro

Makes 10 to 12 servings

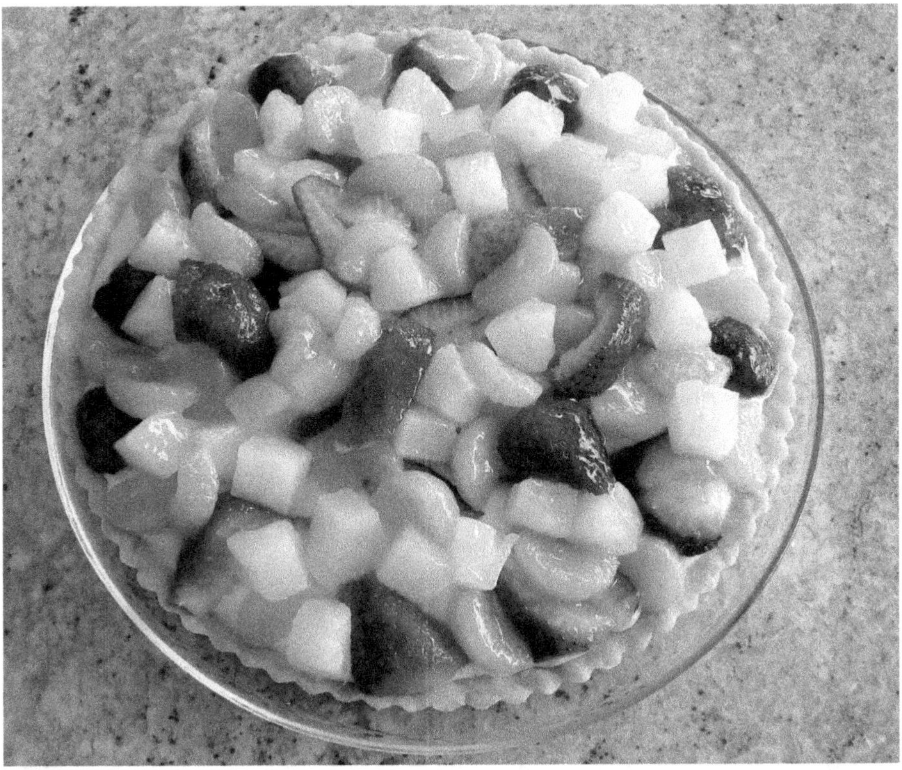

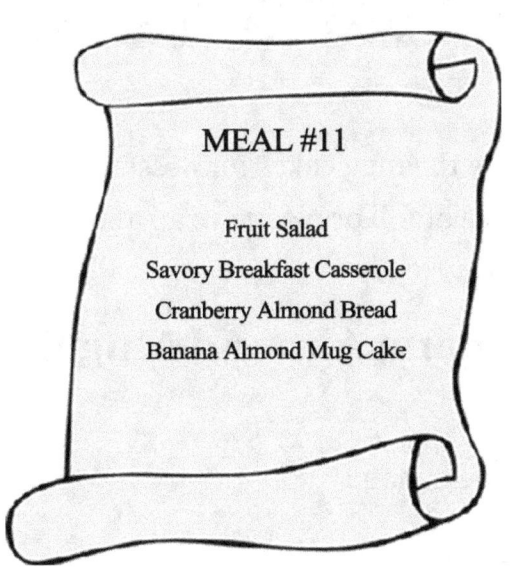

MEAL #11

Fruit Salad

Savory Breakfast Casserole

Cranberry Almond Bread

Banana Almond Mug Cake

Main Grocery Items (Foods like salt, pepper, staples and normal pantry items are not included)

Recipe ingredients have been **totaled** so you can see how much you will need for the entire meal (8 servings).

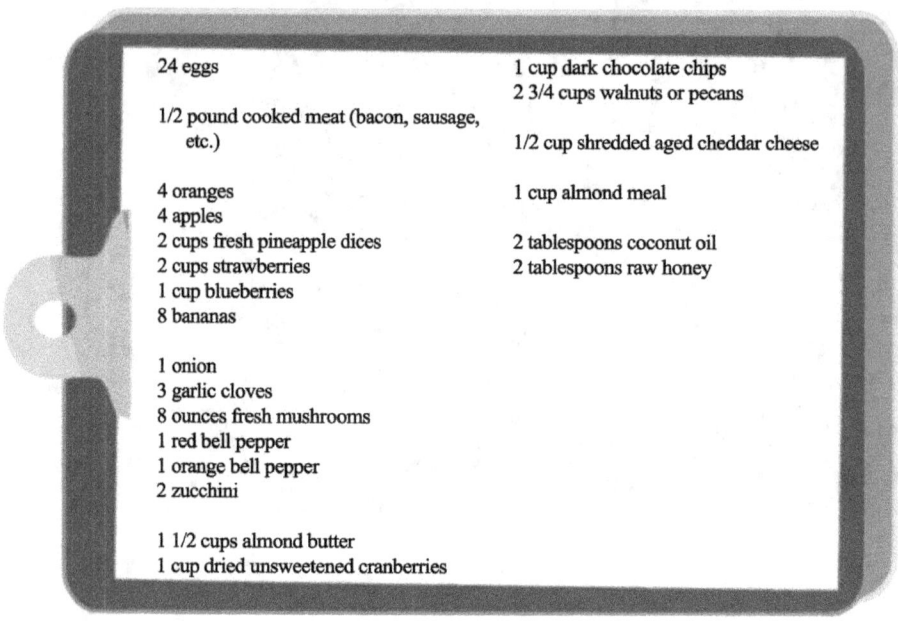

24 eggs	1 cup dark chocolate chips
	2 3/4 cups walnuts or pecans
1/2 pound cooked meat (bacon, sausage, etc.)	
	1/2 cup shredded aged cheddar cheese
4 oranges	1 cup almond meal
4 apples	
2 cups fresh pineapple dices	2 tablespoons coconut oil
2 cups strawberries	2 tablespoons raw honey
1 cup blueberries	
8 bananas	
1 onion	
3 garlic cloves	
8 ounces fresh mushrooms	
1 red bell pepper	
1 orange bell pepper	
2 zucchini	
1 1/2 cups almond butter	
1 cup dried unsweetened cranberries	

Assemble the mug cakes for dessert first. Cover each mug with a piece of foil or plastic wrap and place them into your refrigerator.

Banana Almond Mug Cake

Ingredients:

- 1 very ripe banana

- 1 whole egg

- 2 tablespoons almond butter

- ¼ teaspoon almond extract

- ¼ teaspoon baking soda

- 1/8 teaspoon ground cinnamon

- 2 tablespoons dark chocolate chips

- 2 tablespoons chopped nuts

Directions:

1. Preheat your oven to 350 degree F if you are going to bake it

2. In a ramekin or coffee mug, put the banana and smash it with a fork

3. Now add the egg, almond butter, and extract and mix until the egg is beaten

4. Add in the baking soda, cinnamon, chips and nuts and stir to blend completely

Microwave: Place the mug inside the microwave and process on high for 2 minutes

Oven: Place the mug or ramekin on a baking sheet and bake for 30 minutes

Remove your cake from the oven carefully and enjoy when the cake has had some time to cool and set up

Makes 1 serving

Now that your mug cakes are ready, you will want to get your cranberry almond bread baking in the oven. Once it is cooking, you will want to make your fruit salad and let it chill while you prepare the breakfast casserole.

Cranberry Almond Bread

This bread is moist with zucchini as an ingredient and is heart-healthy with the addition of almond meal and butter. Cranberries, raw honey, nut, and spices also bring lots of flavor to this tasty bread.

Ingredients:

- 4 eggs

- 2 medium zucchini, peeled and grated

- ½ cup almond butter

- 1 cup dried unsweetened cranberries

- 1 cup almond meal

- 2 tablespoons raw honey

- 1½ teaspoons cinnamon

- 1½ teaspoons nutmeg

- 1 teaspoon pumpkin pie spice

- 1 teaspoon baking soda

- ¼ teaspoon sea salt

- ¼ teaspoon ground cloves

- ¾ cup chopped walnuts

Directions:

1. Preheat your oven to 350 degrees F.

2. Prepare a 9" x 5" loaf pan with olive oil spray or apply olive oil with a paper towel.

3. Separate the egg yolks from the egg whites and put each into separate bowls.

4. Beat the egg yolks well.

5. Combine all the remaining ingredients in with the egg yolks, except for the walnuts.

6. Mix all the ingredients well.

7. In a separate bowl, whip the egg whites with an electric beater until they form stiff peaks.

8. Fold in the egg whites with the egg/zucchini mixture.

9. Gently mix in the chopped walnuts.

10. Pour the batter into your greased loaf pan.

11. Bake for 60 minutes until the top is a golden brown color.

12. Test for doneness by inserting a toothpick or cake tester in the center of the bread. It is done when only crumbs appear on the toothpick or tester.

13. Allow the bread to cool for 15-20 minutes before removing it from the pan.

14. Once it is cooled, slice to desired thickness and enjoy.

~~~~~~~~

Fruit Salad

Ingredients:

- 4 oranges peeled and diced, capturing the juice as you prepare them (remove membranes if possible)

- 4 small apples, cored and diced

- 2 cups fresh pineapple dices (capture the juice if preparing dices yourself)

- 2 cups fresh strawberries, sliced

- 1 cup fresh blueberries

- 1 cup walnuts or pecans, chopped (optional)

- 2 teaspoons cinnamon

Directions:

1. In a large serving bowl, combine the oranges with the juice, apples, pineapple with juice, strawberries, and blueberries

2. Add in the nuts

3. Stir gently until thoroughly mixed

4. Sprinkle the top with the cinnamon

Makes 8 servings

~~~~~~~~

Savory Breakfast Casserole

A quick and satisfying dish to start your morning. Using cooked meat and fresh vegetables make this casserole easy to put together.

Ingredients:

- 2 tablespoons coconut oil

- 1 onion, peeled and chopped

- 3 garlic cloves, peeled and minced

- 1 (8 ounce) package fresh sliced mushrooms

- 1 small red bell pepper, seeded and diced

- 1 small orange bell pepper, seeded and diced

- 12 eggs

- ½ pound cooked meat of your choice

- 2 teaspoons each of salt and pepper

- 1 teaspoon paprika

- 1 teaspoon dried thyme

- ½ cup aged shredded cheese for topping (optional)

Directions:

1. Preheat your oven to BROIL

2. Using a large frying pan that can be placed under your broiler, place it on your stovetop and heat up the coconut oil

3. Add the onion and garlic and sauté for 5 minutes to soften the vegetables

4. Add the mushrooms and diced peppers

5. Crack the eggs into a large mixing bowl

6. Add the ingredients except the cheese to the bowl

7. Now pour the egg mixture into the vegetables in the frying pan

8. Stir and allow the eggs to begin to cook on the stove until the sides begin to set

9. Now sprinkle the cheese over the top of the eggs and place the pan under your broiler

10. Cook for approximately 10 minutes to allow the center to finish cooking and the cheese to brown

11. Remove the pan from the broiler and let the pan set for 10 minutes

12. Slice and serve

Makes 8 to 10 servings

As the casserole is finishing up under the broiler, take out your mug cakes from the refrigerator, remove the foil or plastic wrap, set the mugs on a baking tray and put them into a preheated 350 degree F oven. Bake them according to the directions and they will cook while you enjoy your brunch.

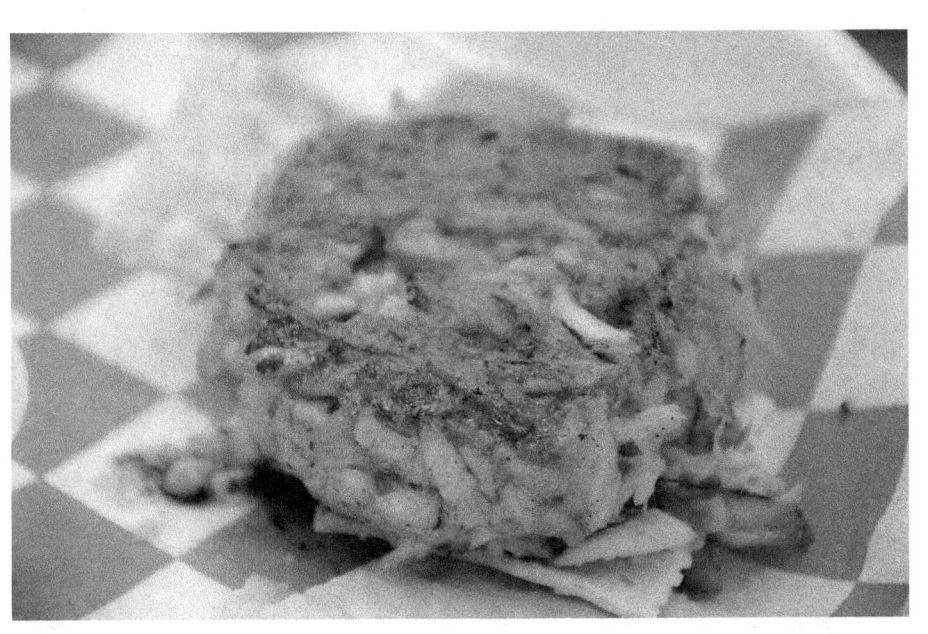

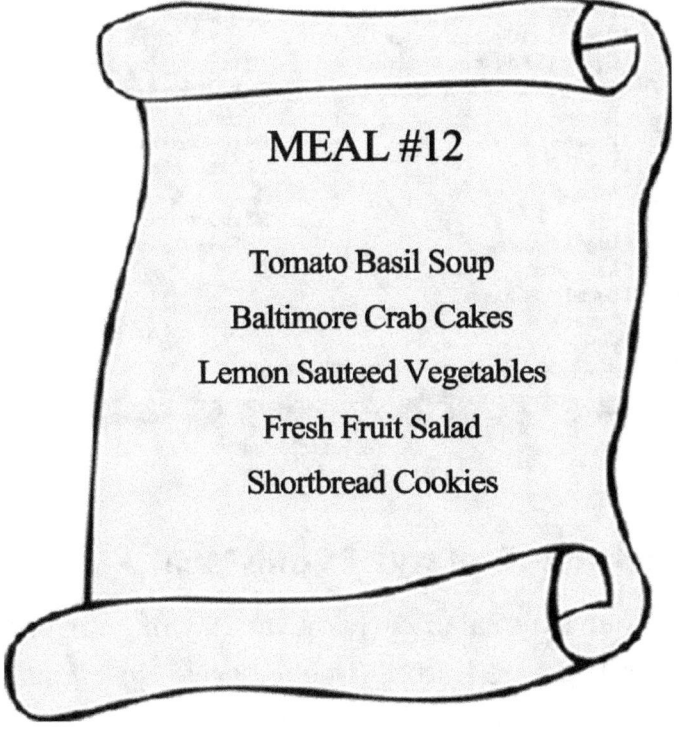

MEAL #12

Tomato Basil Soup

Baltimore Crab Cakes

Lemon Sauteed Vegetables

Fresh Fruit Salad

Shortbread Cookies

This meal is full of seafood goodness and I warn you that it is not a cheap one to make. However, if you want to treat yourself and your friends to a wonderful meal that incorporate food from the sea, this one will definitely fill the bill.

Main Grocery Items (Foods like salt, pepper, staples and normal pantry items are not included)

Recipe ingredients have been **totaled** so you can see how much you will need for the entire meal (8 servings).

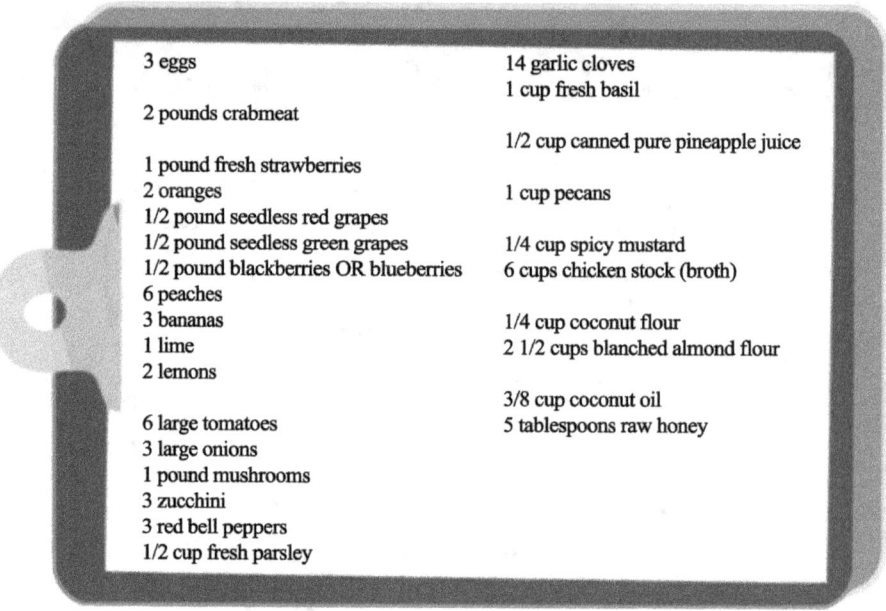

3 eggs	14 garlic cloves
	1 cup fresh basil
2 pounds crabmeat	
	1/2 cup canned pure pineapple juice
1 pound fresh strawberries	
2 oranges	1 cup pecans
1/2 pound seedless red grapes	
1/2 pound seedless green grapes	
1/2 pound blackberries OR blueberries	1/4 cup spicy mustard
6 peaches	6 cups chicken stock (broth)
3 bananas	
1 lime	1/4 cup coconut flour
2 lemons	2 1/2 cups blanched almond flour
	3/8 cup coconut oil
6 large tomatoes	5 tablespoons raw honey
3 large onions	
1 pound mushrooms	
3 zucchini	
3 red bell peppers	
1/2 cup fresh parsley	

 **Early on the Day of Your Meal**

Make your fruit salad early on the day of your party. Then cover and refrigerate it until time to serve. Now would also be a good time to make the dough for your cookies so it can freeze for an hour or so and then you will have time to bake them before lunchtime. (I could suggest you make them the night before but I am afraid there will not be very many left by the time your meal starts).

Also, make up your crab cakes, cover tightly in an airtight container in the refrigerator so they are ready to cook just before time when you are ready to eat them.

Shortbread Cookies

These cookies make a wonderful ending to any meal. Serve with some hot coffee or tea and you will create some wonderful memories.

Ingredients:

- 1 cup pecans, toasted and chopped

- 2½ cups blanched almond flour

- ¼ teaspoon baking soda

- ¼ teaspoon sea salt

- 1 stick salted butter, melted

- 5 tablespoons raw honey, warmed slightly to make it easier to pour

- 1 tablespoon pure vanilla extract

Directions:

1. Preheat your oven to 350 degrees F

2. On a small cookie sheet, place the pecan and cook in your oven for 8 to 10 minutes. Now turn off your oven

3. Remove from the oven and allow to cool, then chop

4. Now place the chopped pecans in a large mixing bowl

5. Add the flour, baking soda, and salt and mix to thoroughly incorporate the soda and salt into the flour

6. In a small separate bowl, add the butter, honey, and vanilla and mix to combine

7. Pour the wet ingredients into the dry ones and mix thoroughly

8. Take a cookie sheet lined with parchment paper and dump the dough out onto it

9. Using your hands, roll the dough back and forth as you form a tube about 2½ to 3 inches in diameter

10. Place the cookie sheet with the dough on it into your freezer for approximately one hour. This will firm up the dough and make it easier to cut into cookies

11. Before removing the dough from the freezer, preheat your oven to 350 degrees F

12. Using a thin knife or dental floss, cut the log into slices. You should get about 24 slices

13. Place the slices on another parchment-lined cookie sheet and bake for approximately 10 minutes. Depending upon the thickness of your slices, you want them to turn a nice golden brown

14. Cool and serve

Makes 20 to 24 cookies

~~~~~~~~

Fresh Fruit Salad

This salad is incredibly tasty, however, you may find it difficult to make it when fruits are out of season. I have used frozen fruit for the peaches, blackberries and blueberries, as well as canned mandarin oranges before and I have been happy with the results. Just make sure you give the fruit plenty of time to defrost and toss very gently when mixing.

Ingredients
- 1 pound strawberries, sliced

- 2 oranges peeled and membrane removed OR 3 large cans mandarin oranges, drained

- ½ pound seedless red grapes, cut in half

- ½ pound seedless green grapes, cut in half

- ½ pound blackberries OR blueberries

- 6 peaches, pitted and cut into chunks

- 3 bananas, peeled and sliced (add just before serving)

- Small amount of raw honey (optional)

Dressing:

- ½ cup pineapple juice

- Juice of one lime

- 1 teaspoon ground cinnamon

Directions:

1. In a large serving bowl, combine the strawberries, oranges, grapes, berries, and peaches

2. Depending upon the sweetness of the fruit, you may want to add a small amount of honey

3. In a small bowl, combine the pineapple juice and lime juice

4. Pour over the fruit and mix gently

5. Place in an airtight container and refrigerate until just before serving

6. Remove from the refrigerator, add the sliced bananas, toss, and sprinkle on the cinnamon

Makes 10 servings

Prepare this soup just before you start cooking the crab cakes and the vegetables. That way it will be all ready in the saucepan and all you will have to do is heat it up just before your meal begins.

Tomato Basil Soup

Ingredients:

- 6 large tomatoes, chopped

- 2 large onion, chopped

- 6 garlic cloves, minced

- 1 tablespoon dried oregano

- 1 teaspoon dried marjoram

- 1 cup fresh basil, coarsely chopped

- 6 cups chicken stock

- Salt and pepper to taste

Directions:

1. Place prepared tomatoes, onions, garlic, oregano, marjoram, and basil into a large saucepan. Add the chicken stock and bring to a boil

2. Reduce the heat and simmer for approximately 20 minutes

3. Cool for 10 minutes

4. Pour the soup into a blender in small batches and run on high for a smooth consistency

5. Repeat for each batch

6. Each time, pour the soup back into another saucepan and reheat briefly before serving

7. Garnish with fresh basil if desired

Makes 8 servings

~~~~~~~~~

Baltimore Crab Cakes

Be sure you have mayonnaise for this recipe. If not, you will want to make that first.

Ingredients:

- 2 pounds crab meat

- ¼ cup coconut flour (or enough to make the mixture stick together)

- 3 eggs

- ½ cup minced fresh parsley

- 4 garlic cloves, minced

- ½ cup Paleolithic mayo

- ¼ cup spicy mustard

- Salt and pepper to taste

- ¼ teaspoon of chipotle powder

- 3–4 tablespoons coconut oil

Directions:

1. If using canned crabmeat, make sure to crumble the crab with your hands into a large mixing bowl and pick out any shells you might find

2. Mix the crab with the coconut flour, egg, parsley, garlic, mayo, mustard, salt, pepper, and chipotle powder

3. In a large skillet, heat the coconut oil over medium heat for about 1 minute

4. Form the crab cake mixture into palm-sized patties and fry for 2–3 minutes on each side or until they are golden brown

Makes enough for 8 people

Just before you start to fry your crab cakes, assemble your vegetable dish. Your stovetop will be a little crowded but the smells will be amazing.

Lemon Sautéed Vegetables

Ingredients:

- 2 tablespoons coconut oil

- 4 garlic cloves, peeled and minced

- 1 medium onion, peeled and finely chopped

- 1 pound mushrooms, sliced

- 3 medium zucchini, peeled and diced

- 3 red bell peppers, seeded and diced

- 8 large basil leaves, thinly sliced

- Juice from 2 lemons

- Sea salt and coarse black pepper to taste

Directions:

1. In a large frying pan, heat the coconut oil

2. When hot, add the garlic, onion, and mushrooms and cook until softened

3. Now add in the zucchini and peppers and cook until softened and heated through

4. Place in a serving bowl and add the basil, lemon juice, salt and pepper

5. Toss gently and serve

Makes 8 servings

Other Resources by Amelia Simons

Gluten-Free Slow Cooker: Easy Recipes for a Gluten Free Diet

Paleolithic Slow Cooker Soups and Stews: Healthy Family Gluten-Free Recipes

Paleolithic Slow Cooker: Simple and Healthy Gluten-Free Recipes

Going Paleolithic: A Quick Start Guide for a Gluten-Free Diet

4 Weeks of Fabulous Paleolithic Breakfasts

4 Weeks of Fabulous Paleolithic Lunches

The Ultimate Paleolithic Collection

4 MORE Weeks of Fabulous Paleolithic Breakfasts

About the Author

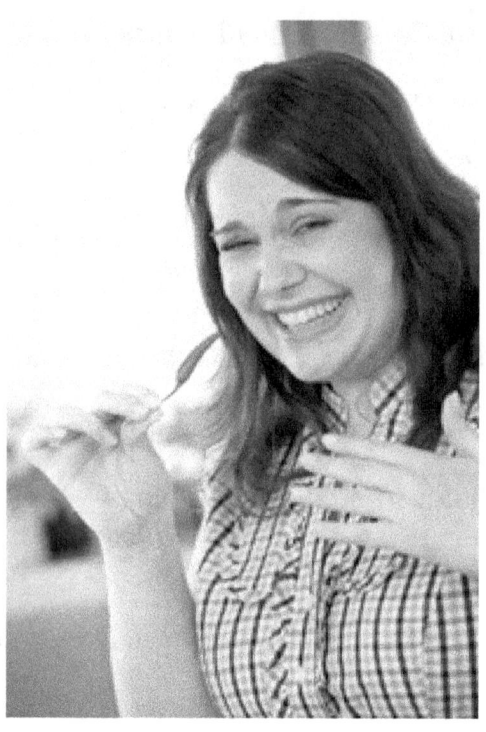

Amelia Simons is a food enthusiast, wife, and mother of five. Frustrated with traditional dieting advice, she stumbled upon the Paleolithic lifestyle of eating and has never looked back. Without bothering to count calories or stress about endless hours of exercise, eating the Paleolithic way enabled Amelia and her husband to effortlessly drop pounds and lower their cholesterol.

Amelia now enjoys sharing the Paleolithic philosophy with friends and readers and finding new ways to turn favorite recipes into healthy alternatives.